New York State Campground Locator Map

New York Campground Map Legend

N — North indicator

→ — Off-map or pinpoint-indication arrow

△ — Campground name and location

Individual tents, platform sites, RV campsites, cabins, lean-tos, and boat access within campground area

△ — Group site

Albany **✪** — Capital

New York **○** — City or town

NATIONAL FOREST STATE PARK — Public lands

Bear Mountain Trl. — Hiking, self-guided, snow-mobile, or biking trails

87 684 — Interstate highways

302 20 6 — U.S. highways

9 28 23A 344 — State roads

Peekamoose Rd. CR 42 — Other roads

Dirt/gravel road

Area boundary

Creek — River or stream

Lake — Ocean, lake, or bay

Amphitheater	Fishing area	Ranger station
Appalachian Trail	Frisbee golf course	Recycle
Basketball court	Golf course	Restroom
Beach	Horse shelter	Sheltered picnic area
Bridge or tunnel	Horse trail	Showers
Cardiac station	Horseshoe pit	Store
Canoe access	Information	Swimming
Dam	Laundry	Telephone
Dining	Marina or boat ramp	Trash disposal
Dump station	Overlook	Tunnel
Electric-access site	Parking	Volleyball court
Firewood	Picnic area	Water
First aid	Pit toilet	Waterfall
Fish-cleaning station	Playground	Wheelchair access

LOCATOR-MAP KEY

BEST TENT CAMPING

NEW YORK STATE

YOUR CAR-CAMPING GUIDE TO SCENIC BEAUTY, THE SOUNDS OF NATURE, AND AN ESCAPE FROM CIVILIZATION

Second Edition

AARON STARMER, CATE STARMER, and TIMOTHY STARMER

MENASHA RIDGE PRESS
Your Guide to the Outdoors Since 1982

**:: *For our parents, who fostered in us a love of the outdoors
and taught us to pitch our first tents.***

Best Tent Camping: New York State

Copyright © 2013 by Aaron Starmer, Cate Starmer, and Timothy Starmer
All rights reserved
Printed in the United States of America
Published by Menasha Ridge Press
Distributed by Publishers Group West
Second edition, first printing

Library of Congress Cataloging-in-Publication Data

    Starmer, Catharine.

    Best tent camping, New York State : your car-camping guide to scenic beauty, the sounds of
nature, and an escape from civilization / Aaron Starmer, Catharine Starmer, Timothy Starmer.
      pages cm. — (Best tent camping)

    Summary: "Wilderness abounds in New York State. From the Great Lakes to the Atlantic Ocean,
from the Adirondack Mountains to the Catskills, from the St. Lawrence River to the Hudson, millions
of acres of public lands are dotted with hundreds of campgrounds—but you probably only have a pre-
cious amount of limited time. Where should you go? When should you go? That's what *Best Tent
Camping: New York State* is for—to help you make the wisest use of your time in the wilds of New York.
Divided geographically into seven sections—Long Island; Catskills and Hudson Valley; Central,
Leatherstocking, and Capital; Adirondacks; Thousand Islands; Finger Lakes; and Western New York—
the book is a helpful reference for camping enthusiasts throughout the state. Historical tidbits,
descriptions of wildlife, and the occasional personal anecdote add flavor to the campground descriptions. Star ratings and maps make choosing the best place to pitch a tent a simple task. Making reservations online or blindly over the phone can put a camper miles from the restroom, stranded with no
shade, or in the middle of a busy campground trail. Maps will help campers avoid those pitfalls, and
wherever possible the authors have even recommended specific campsites for maximum privacy, spaciousness, or beauty." — *Provided by publisher.*

    ISBN-13: 978-0-89732-716-9 (pbk.)
    ISBN-10: 0-89732-716-0 (pbk.)
    ISBN: 978-0-89732-717-6 (ebook); IBN: 978-1-63404-195-9 (hardcover)

    1. Camp sites, facilities, etc.—New York (State)—Guidebooks. 2. Camping—New York (State)—
Guidebooks. 3. New York (State)—Guidebooks. I. Title.

GV191.42.N7S72 2013
917.306809747—dc23

               2013031595

Project editors: Ritchey Halphen and Susan Haynes
Cover design: Scott McGrew
Text design: Annie Long
Cartography: Steve Jones and Scott McGrew
Cover photo: View of North–South Lake and the Hudson Valley (see page 37); © lightphoto
Copyeditor: Susan Cullen Anderson
Proofreader: Lady Vowell Smith
Indexer: Galen Schroeder / dakotaindexing.com

⚜ MENASHA RIDGE PRESS
An imprint of AdventureKEEN
2204 First Avenue South, Suite 102
Birmingham, AL 35233
menasharidge.com

CONTENTS

AUTHORS' TOP NY CAMPGROUNDS

:: BEST FOR HIKING

:: BEST FOR HORSEBACK RIDING

:: BEST FOR PADDLING

:: BEST FOR PRIVACY

:: BEST FOR QUIET

:: BEST FOR SECURITY

:: BEST FOR SPACIOUSNESS

:: BEST FOR SWIMMING

:: BEST FOR WATERFALLS

:: BEST FOR WILDLIFE-VIEWING

ACKNOWLEDGMENTS

We'd like to thank Russell Helms, Ritchey Halphen, Susan Haynes, Larry Bleiberg, Molly Merkle, and the whole gang at Menasha Ridge Press and Keen Communications, whose helpful input and confidence in our abilities saw the first and second editions of this book through to completion.

We started our project nearly seven years ago with a visit to Watch Hill Campground in Long Island, where Marybeth and the staff of the camping concession as well as the rangers of the Fire Island National Seashore confirmed our hope that this project would be hard work but also a lot of fun. Tom Folts and the welcoming staff at the New York State Department of Environmental Conservation made our visits to the Adirondacks and the Catskills especially memorable. The many workers in the New York state-park system always answered our questions with a smile and trusted us enough to set us loose in their facilities with our cameras and notebooks. Finally, we would like to thank our employers for happily tolerating our working vacations, and our friends and families who listened to us blather on about our adventures.

—*Aaron Starmer, Cate Starmer, and Tim Starmer*

PREFACE

We have always been tent campers. From summer nights in the backyard, to family odysseys through the wilds of the Northeast, to trips abroad with pounds of gear strapped to our backs, tent camping has been an essential part of our lives. Did we ever expect to write a book about tent camping? Admittedly, no. But as we loaded up our cars, preparing to take on the task of deciding which 50 places in New York are the best to pitch a tent, we knew we were shouldering a certain responsibility. Choosing a campground can be a frustrating endeavor, a game of dice where you hope your roll won't put you in a glorified parking lot, breathing in exhaust fumes and inserting earplugs to make it through the night. We had to do a good job, because this is a book we ourselves would want to use, many times over.

But New York is a deceptively large state. And there are plenty of campgrounds to go around. Quite early in the project, we discovered we wouldn't have a problem finding worthy candidates. Like coaches, we were faced with the unenviable duty of making cuts. In the Adirondack and Catskill Mountains alone, there are more than 50 state-run campgrounds, to say nothing of privately run facilities and innumerable hike-in sites. We crisscrossed the state, burning up gas, jotting down pages of notes, and, of course, pitching our tents. To our surprise, each campground we visited was quite distinct, and therefore this wouldn't be just a matter of flipping coins.

So we set up a system. We divided the state into seven regions, divisions native New Yorkers will find familiar. We made it a point to provide an even distribution of camping choices. If there were a handful of campgrounds within a few miles of each other, we would choose only the best of the bunch. We favored campgrounds near lakes, rivers, or oceans. We gave preference to surroundings that were either brimming with recreational opportunities or reproduced the quiet thrill of backcountry camping, albeit with the occasional comfort station. Unless the settings were truly spectacular, we shunned campgrounds where RVs were in the majority and reservations were as hard to obtain as those at a fancy restaurant. In short, we chose the campgrounds where we, at different stages in our lives, might find ourselves enjoying a night under the stars.

Maybe you won't find your favorite childhood campground in this book. We hope that what you *will* find are some overlooked campgrounds, located in vibrant (historically, culturally, and naturally) corners of New York. And ideally, you'll get out there to explore as many as possible. We've seen them all, and we can't wait for the next camping season to begin.

INTRODUCTION

When most people think of New York, they naturally think of the Big Apple. While New York City is undoubtedly an essential part of the state, there's so much beyond its borders, especially for those interested in the outdoors. You need travel only a handful of miles north of The Bronx or east of Queens and you will find parks, forests, and beaches where you can spend at least a day and a night. From the Great Lakes to the Atlantic Ocean, from the Adirondack Mountains to the Catskills, from the St. Lawrence River to the Hudson, tent campers wishing to explore the state have a wide variety of campgrounds from which to choose. Here we highlight the 50 best.

Eschewing the noisy, the busy, the overbooked, and the badly maintained, we have chosen peaceful and scenic campgrounds by lakes, on islands, near beaches, along rivers, and deep in the woods.

There are no national parks in New York State, but its state-park system is one of the country's finest. Almost all of the campgrounds featured in this book are state-run and range in size from a dozen campsites to more than 200. Most are accessible by car, but a handful of boat-only and walk-in sites are included for the more adventurous. Most of the parks in the Adirondacks and Catskills are run by the New York State Department of Environmental Conservation, whereas others are run by the New York State Office of Parks, Recreation & Historic Preservation.

The gem of the state's recreational opportunities is easy to spot on a map—a huge patch of green that covers one-fifth of the state: the **Adirondacks.** Conservation of the 6-million-acre Adirondack Park and Forest Preserve has been in effect since 1892, earlier than the creation of almost all the major national parks in the American West. Age is not the only trump card that the Adirondack Park can play: it is larger than Yellowstone, Glacier, Grand Canyon, and Everglades National Parks combined. Parcels of state-owned "forever wild" forests are interspersed with private lands, providing an experience similar to some of the largest parks in Europe. This combination is perfect for tent campers, as the wilderness surrounds you, but supplies and other recreational opportunities always remain nearby. The High Peaks region of the Adirondacks attracts avid hikers, and the innumerable lakes offer something for all types of boats, from large motorboats on Lake George to canoes and kayaks in the St. Regis Canoe Area.

Both the **Catskills** and the **Hudson Valley** have been greatly influenced by their proximity to New York City. The Catskill Park and Forest Preserve is similar to the Adirondacks in its combination of public and private lands (the public portions of the Adirondack and Catskill Parks make up the New York Forest Preserve), but these oldest mountains in the state are known mainly as a playground for the city's wealthy. The Hudson Valley, east of the Catskills, is home to luxurious estates and, of course, the famed river, an essential conduit to and from the bustling metropolis at its mouth.

The heart of New York is the history-rich **Central,** or **Leatherstocking,** region. In addition to Colonial and Revolutionary War sites, visitors will find Howe Caverns and the

Baseball Hall of Fame. We've combined this area with the **Saratoga–Capital** region, home to races of two types: annual horse races in Saratoga Springs and political contests in the capital city of Albany.

The **Finger Lakes,** with their long, thin bodies of water and nearby rolling hills, are remnants from the Ice Ages. Dramatic gorges and waterfalls attract hikers throughout the year, but especially in the spring as floodwaters surge through carved rock walls, and in the fall, when it's a leaf-peeping paradise. More recently, award-winning wineries attract plenty of tourists, including the occasional tent camper.

Long Island is where you will find camping on and near the Atlantic Ocean, perfect for surf fishermen and sun worshipers alike. It may be surprising, but good tent camping can be found not far from the glamorous Hamptons. For a truly unique experience, take the ferry to the car-free Fire Island and its national seashore and pitch your tent in the sand.

Fishing, boating, and water sports attract many visitors to the vacation wonderland known as the **Thousand Islands** on the St. Lawrence River. Getting lost among the myriad islands that form the border between the United States and Canada is a common cruising adventure here. Some people prefer to just relax on the shore and watch ships chug along from America's heartland toward the Atlantic Ocean.

In **Western New York,** the wide shores of Lake Erie flow over Niagara Falls into Lake Ontario. It is also where you'll find the Allegheny Mountains and Allegany State Park, the largest park run by the state's Office of Parks, Recreation & Historic Preservation. Don't miss the deep-cut gorge often referred to as the Grand Canyon of the East, found in Letchworth State Park.

Read on, and we hope that you'll see there is so much more in the state than the skyscrapers and bustling streets of Manhattan. Most upstate natives already know that area is an outdoor destination to rival any in the country, but we believe even the most seasoned New York camper will find some new places to explore. Pitch a tent at any of the campgrounds we feature, and you'll discover even more reasons to love New York.

But before embarking on a trip, take time to prepare. Many of the best tent campgrounds are a fair distance from modern conveniences, and you want to be enjoying yourself rather than making supply or gear runs. Call ahead to each of your selected campgrounds and ask for a park map, brochure, or other information to help you plan your trip. Visit the campground's website (listed under "Key Information" for each destination in this book). Make reservations wherever applicable, especially at popular state parks. Ask questions. Ask more questions. The more questions you ask, the fewer surprises you will encounter. There are other times, however, when you'll want to grab your gear and this book, hop in the car, and just wing it.

:: RESERVATIONS

For all but four of the campgrounds in this book (Adirondak Loj, Peekamoose, Sears Bellows County Park, and Watch Hill), campers should make reservations through **ReserveAmerica**, a convenient online and telephone service that lets you choose from available sites and pay by credit card up to nine months in advance of your stay. For more information, call the

New York State Parks Reservation Center at 800-456-2267, or go to **reserveamerica.com** for 24/7 access.

:: THE OVERVIEW MAP, MAP KEY, AND LEGEND

To find the best campground in a specific part of the state, begin with the overview map, on the inside front cover. It shows you where all 50 of our selected campgrounds are located. The numbers in the diamonds correspond to the campgrounds listed on the facing page.

A map legend that details the symbols found on the campground-layout maps appears on the inside back cover.

:: CAMPGROUND-LAYOUT MAPS

Each profile includes a map showing campsites and facilities. Over the past few years, budget cuts have required the state to reorganize some campgrounds and close others. While we've made every effort to ensure accuracy, note that these maps may not reflect the latest changes.

:: GPS CAMPGROUND-ENTRANCE COORDINATES

Backpackers and campers were among the first outdoorsfolk to adopt GPS technology. Now it seems everyone has a smartphone or a box on their dashboard squawking directions. As GPS tools have become more and more affordable, it makes a lot of sense to include the relevant data in each chapter. Thus, this book provides each campground's location in latitude and longitude, expressed in degrees and decimal minutes. To cover your bases, we also provide street addresses that you can enter into your GPS unit; see "Key Information."

:: THE CAMPGROUND PROFILE

The campground profile is where you will find the nitty-gritty details. Not only is the property described, but readers can get a general idea of the recreational opportunities available— what's in the area and perhaps suggestions for touristy activities.

:: THE FIVE-STAR RATING SYSTEM

This book includes a rating system for New York State's 50 best tent campgrounds. Six campground attributes—beauty, privacy, quiet, cleanliness, security, and spaciousness— are ranked using a five-star system. A low rating in one or two areas, especially privacy and spaciousness, was not necessarily grounds for exclusion from this book. In some cases, the nature of the terrain just doesn't allow for roomy private sites, yet the campground still may be well worth a visit for other qualities. Below and following we describe the criteria for each of the attributes in our five-star rating system:

★ ★ ★ ★ ★   The site is **ideal** in that category.

★ ★ ★ ★   The site is **exemplary** in that category.

★ ★ ★   The site is **very good** in that category.

★ ★   The site is **above average** in that category.

★   The site is **acceptable** in that category.

Beauty

In the best campgrounds, the shapes and elements of nature—flora, water, land, and sky—have melded to create locales that seem to have been made for tent camping. The best sites are so attractive you may be tempted not to leave your outdoor home. A little site work to make the scenic area camper friendly is acceptable, but too many reminders of civilization eliminated many campgrounds from inclusion in this book.

Privacy

A little understory goes a long way toward making you comfortable once you've picked your site for the night. There is a trend toward planting natural borders between campsites if the borders don't already exist. With some trees or brush to define the sites, everyone has personal space, so you can go about the pleasures of tent camping without minding your neighbors.

Quiet

The music of the mountains, rivers, and landscape—the singing birds, rushing streams, and wind whooshing through the trees—includes the kinds of noises tent campers associate with being in outdoors New York. In concert, they camouflage the sounds you don't want to hear—autos coming and going, loud neighbors, and so on.

Cleanliness

Nothing will sabotage a scenic campground like trash. Most of the campgrounds in this guidebook are clean. More-rustic campgrounds—our favorites—usually receive less maintenance. Busy weekends and holidays will show their effects; however, don't let a little litter spoil your good time. Help clean up, and think of it as doing your part for New York's natural environment.

Security

Campground security is relative. A remote campground with no civilization nearby is usually safe, but don't tempt potential thieves by leaving your valuables out for all to see. Use common sense. Campground hosts are wonderful to have around, and state parks with locked gates are ideal for security. Get acquainted with your neighbors and, when possible, develop a buddy system for watching each other's belongings.

Spaciousness

This attribute can be very important, depending on how much of a gearhead you are and the size of your group. Campers with family-style tents need a large, flat spot on which to pitch their tent, but still need to be able to get to the ice chest to access food, while not getting burned by the fire ring. And all of us just want enough room to keep our sleeping, living, and cooking areas separate.

:: WEATHER

Spring is the most variable season for New York State campers. During March, you'll find your first signs of rebirth in the lowlands, yet trees in the high country may not be fully leafed out until June. Both winter- and summerlike weather can occur in spring. As summer approaches, the strong fronts weaken, and thunderstorms and haze become more frequent. Summertime rainy days can be cool. In fall, continental fronts once again sweep through, clearing the air and bringing warm days and cool nights, though rain is always possible.

The first snows of winter usually arrive in November, and snow falls intermittently through April. About 40–120 inches of snow can fall during this time. In winter, expect to experience entire days of below-freezing weather, though the temperatures may range from mild to bitterly cold.

:: FIRST-AID KIT

A useful first-aid kit may contain more items than you might think necessary. These are just the basics. Prepackaged kits in waterproof bags (Atwater Carey and Adventure Medical make them) are available. As a preventive measure, take along sunscreen and insect repellent. Even though quite a few items are listed here, they pack down into a small space:

- Benadryl or the generic equivalent, diphenhydramine (in case of allergic reactions)
- Butterfly-closure bandages
- Epinephrine in a prefilled syringe (EpiPen, for people known to have severe allergic reactions to such outdoor mishaps as bee stings)
- Gauze (one roll)
- Gauze compress pads (six 4-by-4-inch pads)
- Matches or pocket lighter
- Moleskin/Spenco 2nd Skin
- Waterproof first-aid tape
- Whistle (it's more effective in signaling rescuers than your voice)

:: ANIMAL AND PLANT HAZARDS

Snakes

New York has a variety of snakes—including garter, milk, and water snakes—most of which are benign. Timber rattlesnakes, northern copperheads, and Eastern massasauga rattlesnakes are the exceptions, though they primarily dwell in very remote areas. According to the state's Department of Environmental Conservation, the massasauga inhabits two isolated marshy areas: one near Syracuse and the other near Rochester. The copperhead is found mostly along the Hudson Valley but is generally absent from the Catskills. The timber rattler is the most widely dispersed of the three and is found in rugged deciduous forests along the southern edge of the state and up into the eastern Adirondacks. Encounters with any of these species are very rare.

When you hike, stick to well-used trails, and wear over-the-ankle boots and loose-fitting long pants. Rattlesnakes like to bask in the sun and won't bite unless threatened. Don't step or put your hands where you can't see, and avoid wandering in the dark. Step on logs and rocks, never over them (so you can see any snakes on the other side), and be careful when climbing rocks or gathering firewood. Avoid walking through dense brush or willow thickets. Hibernation season is October through April.

Ticks

Ticks are often found on brush and tall grass waiting to hitch a ride on a warm-blooded pass-

Copperhead

Rattlesnake

erby. Adult ticks are most active in New York between April and May and again between October and November. Among the local varieties of ticks, the black-legged tick, commonly called the deer tick, is the primary carrier of Lyme disease. (In general, deer ticks are much smaller than wood, or dog, ticks—about the size of a freckle—and are uniformly dark in color, whereas wood ticks usually have white spots.)

You can use several strategies to reduce your chances of a tick bite. Some people choose to wear light-colored clothing, so ticks can be spotted before they make it to the skin. Most important, be sure to visually check your hair, the back of your neck, your armpits, and your socks at the end of the hike. During your posthike shower, take a moment to do a more complete body check.

For ticks that are already embedded, removal with sharp tweezers is best: place them as close to skin as possible and gently rotate out, taking care not to squeeze the tick. Use disinfectant solution on the wound. To be on the safe side, you may want to visit a physician as soon as possible and follow his or her advice on taking a course of antibiotics to ward off a possible case of Lyme disease. (It takes a few hours for an embedded carrier tick to infect the person it's bitten.)

Poison Ivy, Oak, and Sumac

Recognizing and avoiding these three plants are the most effective ways to prevent the painful, itchy rashes associated with them. Poison ivy *(see photo)* occurs as a vine or ground cover, 3 leaflets to a leaf; poison oak occurs as either a vine or shrub, also with 3 leaflets; and poison

sumac flourishes in swampland, each leaf having 7–13 leaflets.

Urushiol, the oil in the sap of these plants,
is responsible for the rash. Remember that all
parts of the plant contain the oil and you can
get a reaction even from the leafless plant in
winter. Within 14 hours of exposure, raised lines
and/or blisters will appear on the affected area,
accompanied by a terrible itch. Refrain from
scratching, because bacteria under your finger-
nails can cause an infection. Wash and dry the
rash thoroughly, applying a lotion containing

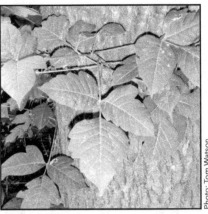

Photo: Tom Watson

calamine to help dry out the rash. If itching or blistering is severe, seek medical attention.

If you do come into contact with one of these plants, remember that oil-contaminated
clothes, pets, or hiking gear can easily cause an irritating rash on you or someone else, so
wash not only any exposed parts of your body but also clothes, gear, and pets.

Black Bears

Black bears live throughout New York, but are most frequently encountered in the Adirondacks and occasionally in the Catskills. Though attacks by black bears are virtually unheard
of, a bear tearing up your gear or rummaging about outside your tent will give anyone a start.
If you encounter a bear at your campsite or while hiking, remain calm and never run away.
Make loud noises to scare off the bear and back away slowly. In primitive and remote areas,
assume that bears are present; in more-developed sites, ask the park staff about the current
bear situation.

Most encounters are food-related, as bears have an exceptional sense of smell and will
eat most anything and everything that you might have in your camping larder. Here are
some important precautions:

- Make sure that your site is clean, and never leave food unattended.

- Store all food, cooking equipment, and garbage in tightly sealed containers
  placed well away from your tent.

- In remote areas or those with recent bear activity, store all items in storage
  lockers or bear canisters, or suspend in a sack 12 feet above the ground, 6 feet
  below branches, and 12 feet from neighboring trees.

- Clean your utensils and cooking equipment at least 100 feet from your site, and
  never dump uneaten food on the ground.

- Do not bring food into your tent.

- Do not sleep in clothes you wore while preparing food.

Generally, proper food preparation and garbage disposal will help maintain a pristine wilderness, ensure the safety of bears and other wildlife, and provide an enjoyable camping experience for everyone.

:: TIPS FOR A HAPPY CAMPING TRIP

There is nothing worse than a bad camping trip, especially because it is so easy to have a great time. To assist with making your outing a rewarding one, here are some pointers:

- Reserve your site ahead of time, especially if it's a weekend or holiday, or if the campground is wildly popular. Many prime campgrounds require at least a six-month lead time on reservations. **Check before you go.**

- Pick your camping buddies wisely. A family trip is pretty straightforward, but you may want to reconsider including grumpy Uncle Fred, who doesn't like bugs, sunshine, or marshmallows. After you know who's going, make sure that everyone is on the same page regarding expectations of difficulty (amenities or the lack thereof, physical exertion, and so on), sleeping arrangements, and food requirements.

- Don't duplicate equipment such as cooking pots and lanterns among campers in your party. Carry what you need to have a good time, but don't turn the trip into a major moving experience.

- Dress for the season. Check the temperature highs and lows of the area you plan to visit during the time of year you will be there. It may be warm at night in the summer in your backyard, but up in the mountains it will be quite chilly.

- Pitch your tent on a level surface, preferably one covered with leaves, pine straw, or grass. Use a tarp or specially designed footprint to thwart ground moisture and to protect the tent floor. Do a little site maintenance, such as picking up the small rocks and sticks that can damage your tent floor and make sleep uncomfortable. If you have a separate tent rain fly but don't think you'll need it, keep it rolled up at the base of the tent in case it starts raining at midnight.

- If you are not comfortable sleeping with just the tent floor between you and the ground, take a sleeping pad with you that is full-length and thicker than you think you might need. This not only will keep your hips from aching on hard ground but also will help keep you warm. A wide range of thin, light, inflatable pads is available at camping stores today, and these are a much better choice than home air mattresses, which conduct heat away from the body and tend to deflate during the night.

- Unless you are hiking to a primitive campsite, there is no real need to skimp on food due to weight. Plan tasty meals and bring everything you will need to prepare, cook, eat, and clean up.

■ If you tend to use the bathroom multiple times at night, you should plan ahead. Leaving a warm sleeping bag and stumbling around in the dark to find the restroom, whether it be a pit toilet, a fully plumbed comfort station, or just the woods, is not fun—nor is it safe from unexpected wildlife encounters. Keep a flashlight and any other accoutrements you may need by the tent door and know exactly where to head in the dark.

■ Standing dead trees and storm-damaged living trees can pose a real hazard to tent campers. These trees may have loose or broken limbs that could fall at any time. When choosing a campsite or even just a spot to rest during a hike, *look up.*

:: CAMPING ETIQUETTE

Camping experiences can vary wildly depending on a variety of factors, such as weather, preparedness, fellow campers, and time of year. Here are a few tips on creating good vibes with fellow campers and wildlife you encounter:

■ Obtain all required permits and authorization. Make sure you check in, pay your fee, and mark your site as directed. Don't make the mistake of grabbing a seemingly empty site that looks more appealing than your site. It could be reserved. If you're unhappy with the site you've selected, check with the campground host for other options.

■ Leave only footprints. Be sensitive to the ground beneath you. Be sure to place all garbage in designated receptacles or pack it out if none is available. No one likes to see the trash someone else has left behind.

■ Never spook animals. It's common for animals to wander through campsites, where they may be accustomed to the presence of humans (and food). An unannounced approach, a sudden movement, or a loud noise startles most animals. A surprised animal can be dangerous to you, to others, and to themselves. Give them plenty of space.

■ Plan ahead. Know your equipment, your ability, and the area where you are camping—and prepare accordingly. Be self-sufficient at all times; carry necessary supplies for changes in weather or other conditions. A well-executed trip is a satisfaction to you and to your fellow campers.

■ Be courteous to campers, hikers, bikers, and others you encounter.

■ Strictly follow the campground's rules regarding the building of fires. Never burn trash. Trash smoke smells horrible and is often toxic, and trash debris in a fire pit or grill is unsightly.

:: BACKCOUNTRY-CAMPING ADVICE

A permit is not required before entering the backcountry to camp in the Adirondacks and Catskills. However, you should practice low-impact camping. Adhere to the adages "Pack it in, pack it out" and "Take only pictures, leave only footprints." **Leave No Trace** camping ethics are essential while in the backcountry (see **lnt.org** for more information).

Open fires are permitted except during dry times, when the forest service may issue a fire ban. Backpacking stoves are strongly encouraged. You are required to hang your food away from bears and other animals to prevent them from becoming introduced to (and dependent on) human food. Wildlife learns to associate backpacks and backpackers with easy food sources, thereby influencing animal behavior.

Solid human waste must be buried in a hole at least 3 inches deep and at least 200 feet away from trails and water sources; a trowel is basic backpacking equipment.

Following the previous guidelines will increase your chances for a pleasant, safe, and low-impact interaction with nature.

:: VENTURING AWAY FROM THE CAMPGROUND

If you go for a hike, bike, or other excursion into the wilderness, here are some tips:

- Always carry food and water, whether you are planning to go overnight or not. Bring potable water or treat water by boiling or filtering before drinking from a lake or stream.

- Stay on designated trails, but if you become disoriented, don't panic. As soon as you think you may be off-track, stop, assess your current direction, and then retrace your steps back to where you went awry. If you have absolutely no idea how to continue, even from that awry point, return to the trailhead the way you came in. Should you become completely lost and have no idea of how to return to the trailhead, remaining in place along the trail and waiting for help is most often the best option for adults and always the best option for children.

- Be especially careful when crossing streams. Whether you are fording the stream or crossing by stepping on a log, make every step count. If you have any doubt about maintaining your balance on a log, go ahead and ford the stream instead. When fording a stream, use a trekking pole or stout stick for balance and face upstream as you cross. If a stream seems too deep to ford, turn back.

- Be careful at overlooks. Although these areas may provide spectacular views, they are potentially hazardous. Stay back from the edge of outcrops and be absolutely sure of your footing—that the ground beneath you is stable and not subject to crumbling rock or dirt. A misstep can mean a nasty and possibly fatal fall.

- Know the symptoms of hypothermia. Shivering and forgetfulness are the two most common indicators of this insidious killer, which can strike even in summer. To prevent it, dress in layers: wear synthetic clothing (not cotton) for insulation, don a cap and gloves to reduce heat loss, and protect yourself with waterproof, breathable outerwear. If symptoms arise, seek shelter, a fire, hot liquids, and dry clothes or a dry sleeping bag.

Long
Island

1

Sears Bellows County Park

Pitch a tent in the calm, wooded surroundings of
Long Island's pinelands.

When we told our friends that we would be spending some time camping on Long Island, we were met with blank stares. "Who on Long Island ever goes camping?" was a common question. Evidently, a lot of people. Suffolk County alone has 11 campgrounds in its park system. We found the best of the lot, as far as tent camping goes, at Sears Bellows County Park. With attractive ponds, bridle paths, and hiking trails, the park is a pleasant enclave just west of the Hamptons, and the campground features something that is rare these days—a tent-only section.

To regulate use of its 48,000 acres of parkland, Suffolk County has instituted a system called the Green Key. Forget about trying to use your Empire Passport or booking through ReserveAmerica. In Suffolk, the Green Key rules are more than a little complex. The Green Key is a pass (valid for three years) that county residents must purchase in order to qualify for reduced fees at county parks, as well as access to the golf course and campground-reservation system. Non-residents can purchase a Tourist Green Key, which extends many of the same privileges,

but it is more expensive and lasts only a year. Suffolk County residents probably already know all about this, but for more information on the byzantine rules explaining the procurement and use of the mighty key, call 631-854-4949, or visit the Suffolk County website, **suffolkcountyny.gov.**

Once you have a Green Key, you're ready to start camping. And for tent campers, Sears Bellows is a good place to start. The park is not situated on the Atlantic or Long Island Sound, like most parks where RVs are the name of the game. It's inland, wedged at the bottleneck of land where the south fork of Long Island splits off. You can't play golf or water-ski here (or drink a beer, for that matter), but you can pitch a tent in the calm, wooded surroundings of Long Island's pinelands.

The campground's two loops are set off diagonally from each other and are split by the main park road. The trailer-only loop and group-camping sections are found just past the park office, to the right. Farther down the road and to the left is the tent-only section. There are 30 sites to choose from here, and all are relatively flat and surrounded by towering pines. If you are reserving online, the site informs you which sites have more shade. The exterior sites are generally more private, but the most isolated one we found was 23, an interior site.

Water spigots are well distributed, but if you're camping on the outer edge of the

:: Ratings

BEAUTY: ★ ★
PRIVACY: ★ ★
QUIET: ★ ★ ★
CLEANLINESS: ★ ★
SECURITY: ★ ★ ★
SPACIOUSNESS: ★ ★ ★

:: Key Information

ADDRESS: Bellows Pond Road, Hampton Bays, NY 11946

OPERATED BY: Suffolk County Department of Parks, Recreation and Conservation

CONTACT: 631-852-8290 and 631-244-7275; suffolkcountyny.gov

OPEN: Early April–late May (Thursday–Saturday); late May–early September (all week)

SITES: 70 (30 tent-only, 40 trailer-only)

SITE AMENITIES: Picnic table and fire ring

ASSIGNMENT: Choose from available sites

REGISTRATION: On arrival or by reservation

FACILITIES: Water, flush toilets, showers, pay phone

PARKING: At site, maximum 2 vehicles

FEE: $15/night (Resident Green Key); $30/night (Tourist Key); $12 reservation fee

ELEVATION: 20'

RESTRICTIONS:

■ **Pets:** Dogs on leash with proof of currently valid rabies vaccination; 2 pets maximum/site

■ **Fires:** In fire rings only

■ **Alcohol:** No alcohol permitted

■ **Vehicles:** No limit

■ **Other:** Quiet hours 10 p.m.–8 a.m.

■ **Reservations:** No minimum stay required

loop, you will have a short walk downhill to the comfort station. Overall, the accommodations are a bit rustic and, when we visited, could have used some more upkeep. Sites here are, however, a welcome change from the paved and cluttered ones you find elsewhere in the county. You feel as if you are in the thick of the woods, even though the suburbs are not far away.

You can catch a glimpse of Bellows Pond from some of the sites, but none could be considered waterfront. Still, it's a quick hop down to the shores of Bellows, where you can go swimming at the beach from early June to Labor Day (when lifeguards are on duty) or grab a fishing pole, rent a rowboat, and try for some bluegill, bass, perch, and pickerel. You'll find a small activity field not far from the sites, but most people will want to spend more time at the beach or at the picnic pavilion and playground, both of which have great views. Reservations can be made for group events, and a large corner of the park across the water from the campground has been set off for this purpose. Many youth groups come to Sears Bellows during the summer for camping, picnicking, and games.

Strap on your boots, take off on some of the trails, and visit some of the park's other ponds. There are the Munn's Ponds, along with Grass, Little House, Big House, and Division Ponds, to say nothing of Sears Pond, the largest of the bunch. The longest hiking trail, about 3 miles round-trip, leaves directly from the campground, crosses over bridle trails, and loops around shores of Sears. As for the bridle trails, they can be explored on horseback by shelling out a few dollars at the Sears Bellows Stables, which is on the northern edge of the park, right next to the Big Duck.

What is the Big Duck, you ask? Suffolk County calls it "Long Island's most famous

1 Sears Bellows County Park Campground

landmark," and it is listed in the National Register of Historic Places. Basically, it's a gift shop and information booth in the shape of a giant white duck. Built during the 1930s, it was for many years a store that sold (what else?) ducks. In 1987, the structure was donated to the state, and since then it has served as a retailer of Long Island memorabilia (most of it duck-themed) and a provider of tourist information. Hearing of this beloved monument, we imagined a towering roadside oddity but were a bit let down to see that it's smaller than some of today's RVs. But do stop by during your visit to Sears Bellows and learn a bit about the region. Chances are you will be surprised by the many outdoor adventures to be found in Suffolk County.

:: Getting There

Follow NY 27 (Sunrise Highway) to Exit 65. Take NY 24 North 1.5 miles and turn left on Bellows Pond Road. The park entrance is on the right.

GPS COORDINATES   N40° 53.750'   W72° 33.183'

2

Watch Hill

At night, you will probably hear only the soft chatter of other campers, the gentle sounds of the wind and wildlife, and, on especially quiet evenings, the roar of the ocean.

New York State has no national parks. However, just off the coast of Long Island is Fire Island National Seashore (operated by the National Park Service), a string of small communities connected by miles of undeveloped beach. At Watch Hill Campground, within the national seashore, you'll find some of the best tent camping in the state. With 26 walk-in sites situated among the dunes no more than 50 yards from the ocean, it distinguishes itself as a campground that promises beach camping and actually delivers.

No roads run the length of Fire Island. Raised boardwalks above the dunes and marshes are the thoroughfares. Golf carts provide speedy travel for maintenance workers. Little red wagons (think Radio Flyers) serve as pack mules for groceries and supplies. No roads mean no cars and certainly no RVs. This makes getting to the island a little complicated, but it's worth the effort. May–October, there is regular ferry service to Watch Hill from Patchogue, New York, with peak service (four to six departures per day) during summer months. Be sure to check **davisparkferry.com** for an exact schedule, as it changes from month to month.

Upon reaching the island, the extensive marina serves as your jumping-off point. The park provides slips for visiting boaters, but don't worry about motor-related noise. The campground is still a quarter-mile away. At the marina you'll find the Watch Hill Visitor Center and Ranger Station, the dock shack (where campers check in), and a small store. When we visited, a snack bar and a popular dockside restaurant were also open. In October 2012, Hurricane Sandy permanently changed the landscape and damaged many buildings on the island. At the time of this writing recovery efforts were just under way, so the exact layout and some amenities will have most likely changed by the time you read this, but rest assured that the windswept beauty will remain intact.

The campground is a short walk from the marina, so a sturdy backpack to carry supplies would be useful. No ground fires are allowed at sites, but each is equipped with a grill, and you'll definitely want to bring a bag of charcoal. You'll also want to load up on insect repellent and sunscreen. In the summer, mosquitoes are thick; shrubs protect the sites from the wind, but there is little natural shade.

:: Ratings

BEAUTY: ★ ★ ★ ★ ★
PRIVACY: ★ ★ ★ ★
QUIET: ★ ★ ★ ★
CLEANLINESS: ★ ★ ★ ★
SECURITY: ★ ★ ★ ★
SPACIOUSNESS: ★ ★ ★

:: Key Information

ADDRESS: Watch Hill Ferry Terminal, Patchogue, NY 11772; P.O. Box 4, Sayville, NY 11782

OPERATED BY: Fire Island Concessions

CONTACT: 631-567-6664; watchhillfi.com

OPEN: Mid-May–mid-October

SITES: 26 individual sites (including 1 that is wheelchair-accessible); 1 group site; backcountry camping available through the National Park Service, 631-597-6455

SITE AMENITIES: Picnic table and grill

ASSIGNMENT: Choose from available sites

REGISTRATION: On arrival

FACILITIES: Water, flush toilets, showers, marina store

PARKING: At ferry station only

FEE: $25/night

ELEVATION: 4'

RESTRICTIONS:

■ **Pets:** Dogs on leash with proof of currently valid rabies vaccination

■ **Fires:** In grill only

■ **Alcohol:** At site

■ **Vehicles:** None permitted; all sites are walk-in

■ **Other:** Check in 10 a.m.–4 p.m.; quiet hours 10 p.m.–6 a.m.; 8-person limit (no more than 5 adults); swimming only with certified lifeguard; carry out all trash

■ **Reservations:** 2-night stay required for weekends

Boardwalks connect the campground amenities, and buildings are raised to protect the dunes. The main boardwalk winds its way east from the marina to a comfort station with flush toilets and showers. One path continues south over the dunes, to the beach, while a narrower path leads east, directly to the campground. The wheelchair-accessible, group, and host sites are the first ones you pass. The remaining sites are well distributed along the boardwalk, which is lined with fire extinguishers, water spigots, and one wash station.

When you arrive at Watch Hill, site selection is first come, first served. We recommend sites 2, 10, 25, and 26 for their privacy and distance from the boardwalk. Campsites not directly connected to the boardwalk can be accessed along sandy paths through other sites. The boardwalk through the camping area is popular with day visitors, often families exploring the area or local residents out jogging. At night, the only sounds you'll hear are the soft chatter of other campers, the gentle sounds of the wind and wildlife, and, on especially quiet evenings, the roar of the ocean.

Reservations are available exclusively online through **watchhillfi.com.** If you would like to spend the night beyond the confines of the campground, backcountry-camping permits are available only through the National Park Service. There are many rules and regulations, and you will want to contact the Watch Hill Visitor Center for more details. Backcountry campers should be particularly careful about ticks and poison ivy.

Spend some time exploring the raised nature trail that climbs within the nearby narrow forest and provides great views of your tent before winding through the marshy northern side of the island. The Great South Bay spreads out before you, with the southern shore of Long Island, 4 miles away, usually visible. Keep an eye out for deer, rabbits, shorebirds, and other coastal creatures.

2 Watch Hill Campground

Rangers conduct interpretive programs during the summer that introduce even more hidden wildlife. A guided canoe trip is an enjoyable way to explore the area's salt marshes and tidal ecosystem. And a jaunt to Davis Park, a charming community of seasonal homes a mile west of the campground, is always recommended.

The beach, understandably, attracts the most visitors. Follow the boardwalk to the beach to enjoy the sights, sounds, and smells of the Atlantic. Swimming is allowed only when lifeguards are present in summer. Watch for sections of beach roped off to protect the nesting areas of the federally protected piping plover. Be careful to stay off the dunes to preserve Fire Island for future visitors. Respecting this fragile barrier island will ensure it stays a summer destination for many generations.

:: Getting There

From I-495, take Exit 63 to North Ocean Avenue (CR 83). Follow North Ocean Avenue south 4 miles to Patchogue. Turn right onto Montauk Highway (NY 27A). Take the next left onto West Avenue. Drive one block. The parking lot for the Watch Hill Ferry Terminal is on the right.

**GPS COORDINATES
(WATCH HILL MARINA ENTRANCE)**   N40° 41.533'   W72° 59.417'

3

Wildwood State Park

While heavily wooded, the park also contains an attractive beach bordered with steep, windswept bluffs.

When the sun comes out and tourists are heading to the Hamptons or Fire Island, it is easy to forget the North Fork of Long Island and its distinctive charms. At the western edge of the North Fork, nestled between a patchwork of farmland and Long Island Sound, you will find Wildwood State Park. With its extensive campground, it is an ideal place to begin your explorations of the region, or to simply spend some time hiking and relaxing near the beach.

At 600 acres, Wildwood has a lot to offer for a small state park. Its distinct advantages over most other parks are that it is heavily wooded and has an attractive beach bordered by steep, windswept bluffs. This combination keeps a steady stream of visitors—especially campers—coming and going throughout the summer.

The park itself may be small, but the campground is the largest on Long Island. The 242 tent sites can fill quickly, so reservations are recommended on weekends and holidays. At other times, walk-ins should be easily accommodated.

:: Ratings

BEAUTY: ★ ★ ★ ★
PRIVACY: ★ ★ ★
QUIET: ★ ★ ★
CLEANLINESS: ★ ★ ★ ★
SECURITY: ★ ★ ★
SPACIOUSNESS: ★ ★ ★ ★

When you enter the campground and register at the camp office, you will see a large RV-camping area. Fortunately for tent campers, the park has separated these 80 electric-equipped sites from the more-remote tent sites. After registering, simply bear left from the office and follow the signs to the five tenting loops. You will enter Loop B first. In the spring and autumn months, only Loops B and D are open. After Memorial Day, all loops are open. Loops A and C are sandwiched in the middle of the campground. Loop E forms the far border and offers the most private camping experience.

All sites are wooded and well spaced. Naturally, sites along the outside edge of the loops are more secluded, but are also farthest from the comfort stations. If you need a flat and dry surface on which to pitch your tent, try Loop C. Equipped with a number of wooden tent platforms—available for an extra charge—Loop C is the most "civilized" of the loops. Some of the more spacious and private sites include C1, C19, D14, E24, and E25.

All sites lack both fire rings and grills. Fires are allowed, but only in approved containers with metal sides and bottoms. You can bring your own, but we recommend renting one from the campground vendor. Quiet hours are from 10 p.m. to 7 a.m. Even though the RV section is removed from the tents, all campers will appreciate that generators are also prohibited during this time. Because of the campground's size, enforcing quiet hours

:: Key Information

ADDRESS: Hulse Landing Road, P.O. Box 518, Wading River, NY 11792

OPERATED BY: New York State Office of Parks, Recreation and Historic Preservation

CONTACT: 631-929-4314; nysparks.com/parks/68/details.aspx

OPEN: Early April–early October

SITES: 314 (80 electrical hookups)

SITE AMENITIES: Picnic table

ASSIGNMENT: Choose from available sites or reservations

REGISTRATION: On arrival

FACILITIES: Water, flush toilets, showers, dump station, camp store

PARKING: At site, 1 vehicle maximum, 1 additional car at separate lot for fee

FEE: $15–$18/night (plus $4/night on Fridays, Saturdays, and holidays)

ELEVATION: 167'

RESTRICTIONS:

▨ **Pets:** Not allowed

▨ **Fires:** In approved containers only (available for rent at campground office)

▨ **Alcohol:** Prohibited

▨ **Vehicles:** Up to 50'

▨ **Other:** Quiet hours 10 p.m.–7 a.m.

▨ **Reservations:** 2-night stay required

isn't always the easiest task for the accommodating staff. But also because of its size, there are plenty of spots to find solitude.

Once you've established camp at Wildwood, take time to explore the North Fork of Long Island. Kids will probably beg to make a stop at Splish-Splash Water Park in Riverhead. The older crowd might find touring the many wineries that dot NY 25 more to their pace. Take the scenic drive out to Greenport to catch the ferry to Shelter Island, or continue on to Orient Beach State Park at the far eastern end of the fork.

If you choose to stay in the park, you'll still find plenty to do. During summer months, the campground offers movies, children's theater, square dancing, and magic and wildlife shows. A fall festival is an annual event.

To enjoy some quiet time away from the campground, take to the 12 miles of color-coded hiking and biking trails that circle and bisect the park. Nearly three-fourths of this land is undeveloped hardwood forest. One of the most popular hikes starts where the

Pedestrian Walk meets the beach parking lot. The trail meanders for nearly 4 miles, opening onto the bluffs and lovely views of Long Island Sound.

The beach itself is a short stroll from the campground along the Pedestrian Walk, but some campers choose to drive to the closer visitor lot. A large picnic area, playground, and concession stands border the lot, shaded throughout by tall trees. During the summer, this day-use area attracts plenty of local visitors, who pack up the family and walk down the steep, paved path to the beach.

A bathhouse (with another concession stand) sits squarely in the center of the beach, but the main draw is the water and the beauty of the bluffs. The high, sandy bluffs slope down to a narrow beach and rolling waves. Because of erosion, the bluffs, with their delicate vegetation, are strictly off-limits. The beach stretches in both directions, with fishing and bathing areas clearly designated. You can walk for miles, but if

3 Wildwood Campground

you just want to take it easy, spreading out a towel and looking out onto Long Island Sound is an appealing option.

According to one campground worker, "lots of city folks" come out each summer. But because of the range of activities offered and the appealing combination of forest and beach on display, the campground attracts people of all stripes, including that same employee, who told us that he planned to spend his vacation time camping with friends at Wildwood.

:: Getting There

From I-495, take Exit 68 to NY 46 North. Follow NY 46 North 7 miles to NY 25A East. Turn left onto Sound Avenue. Turn left at the traffic light onto Hulse Landing Road. The park entrance is on the right.

GPS COORDINATES N40° 57.750' W72° 48.550'

Catskills and Hudson Valley

4

Clarence Fahnestock Memorial State Park

Fahnestock is distinguished by roads that twist around large seams of stone jutting up among the trees.

For the 88 miles it passes through New York State, the Appalachian Trail meanders over relatively flat, wooded terrain, never rising past 1,500 feet. For some, it is one of the least memorable sections of the trail. More than 10 miles of the route, however, passes through Clarence Fahnestock Memorial State Park, a 12,000-acre gem with some of the best hiking in the Hudson Highlands. And just a few hundred yards from the famed trail is an attractive campground, nestled into one of the park's many ridges.

Along the scenic Taconic State Parkway and only 60 miles from New York City, Fahnestock, as it is commonly called, attracts plenty of visitors looking for short day hikes. There are plenty of brief rambles to experience, but the tent camper will discover that the park deserves at least a few days of exploration. Not only does it serve as a jumping-off (or stopping-off) point on the Appalachian Trail, it also features seven small mountains to summit, a series of

attractive lakes and ponds, horse and bike paths, and a good-size beach for summertime swimming.

For us, the campground alone was worth the visit. While many campgrounds are no more than wooded parking lots, the one at Fahnestock is distinguished by roads that twist around large seams of stone jutting up among the trees. Tucked into the rock outcrops, the sites offer more isolation from neighbors than one might expect and are surprisingly flat compared to the surrounding terrain. The first section (1–29) includes a series of walk-in sites set about 30 yards from the road. It is a short distance, but with many of the cars for these sites parked along the camp road, it can at least give the illusion that you are "packing it in."

Sites 25 and 30, perched among the rocks and well shaded, are among the most desirable. The most spacious sites, numbered 30–50, are those spread along the edge of the looping road. Inside the loop, grassy lots essentially serve as sites 51–68. Another jumble of sites (70–81) sits in a grassy lot near Pelton Pond. The only good reason to stay in these crowded lots is if you are booking connecting multiple sites. Two comfort stations serve opposite ends of the campground. Though all sites are technically open to trailers, it's unlikely that you'll see one. There are no hookups or dumping stations for RVs.

:: Ratings

BEAUTY: ★ ★ ★ ★
PRIVACY: ★ ★ ★ ★
QUIET: ★ ★ ★ ★
CLEANLINESS: ★ ★
SECURITY: ★ ★ ★
SPACIOUSNESS: ★ ★ ★ ★

:: Key Information

ADDRESS: 1498 NY 301, Carmel, NY 10512

OPERATED BY: New York State Office of Parks, Recreation and Historic Preservation

CONTACT: 845-225-7207; nysparks.com/parks/133

OPEN: Late April–early December

SITES: 79

SITE AMENITIES: Picnic table, grill, and fire ring

ASSIGNMENT: Choose from available sites or reservations

REGISTRATION: On arrival

FACILITIES: Water, pit and flush toilets, showers

PARKING: At site, maximum 2 vehicles

FEE: $15/night (plus $4/night on Fridays, Saturdays, and holidays)

ELEVATION: 1,059'

RESTRICTIONS:

■ **Pets:** Dogs on leash with proof of currently valid rabies vaccination

■ **Fires:** In fire rings or grills only

■ **Alcohol:** At site

■ **Vehicles:** Up to 30'

■ **Other:** Quiet hours 10 p.m.–7 a.m.; Swimming only in Canopus Lake when lifeguard present (weekends in June, daily in July and August); no gas motors in Canopus Lake; no swimming or boats in Pelton Pond

■ **Reservations:** 2-night stay required

Pelton Pond, a small body of water at the edge of the campground, is a great spot to cast a fishing line. Neither swimming nor boating is allowed, but the pond is regularly stocked with rainbow trout. Nearby John Allen Pond and Canopus Lake are also chock-full of bass, perch, and sunfish. Anglers must obtain a New York State fishing license before cracking open their tackle boxes. And those wishing to fish the park's Stillwater Lake must obtain an additional permit from the park office.

The park's Taconic Education Center is mainly for reserved group use, but the nature center at the northern point of Pelton Pond offers interpretive programs on summer weekends. The 1.5-mile Pelton Pond Nature Trail is a nice little loop that will introduce visitors to the flora and fauna of the area. But the white blazes of the Appalachian Trail are what will draw a large number of hikers. A 5-mile segment of the trail can be followed from the south end of Canopus Lake up along a ridge to great views of the area. One of the park's brochures recommends doing the hike in June, when the mountain laurels are in bloom.

You may choose from more than 42 miles of trails in the park. Anglers will want to take the 5-mile Three Lakes Hike, which showcases the three larger fishing spots mentioned above and follows a former mine-railroad path. The region was mined for iron ore for nearly 100 years, ending in 1876, when competition got the best of the local industry. A Manhattan doctor named Clarence Fahnestock purchased sections of what is now the park in the early 20th century. He died during World War I in France, and his family donated the land to the state in his memory.

After a day of hiking, the spring-fed Canopus Lake and its large man-made beach offer a refreshing respite. The soft white sand attracts many bathers and is extremely popular for day-use visitors; campers enjoy free access and may bring two cars to the parking

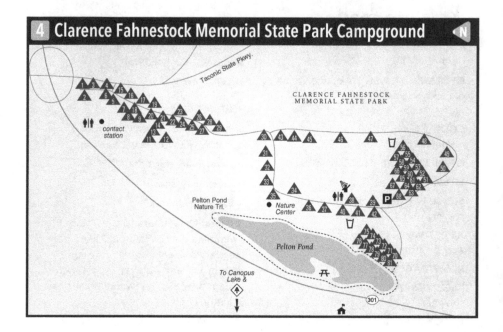

lot. There's a concession stand, showers, grills, swimming, boat rentals, and more—certainly enough to keep campers busy and cool on a hot summer day.

:: Getting There

From Taconic State Parkway, take NY 301 West 0.25 mile to the park entrances.

GPS COORDINATES   N41° 27.950'   W73° 49.500'

5

Devil's Tombstone

The satanic nomenclature is still appropriate today, as this is the jumping-off point for one of the most grueling hikes in the Catskills: the Devil's Path Trail.

Traditional Dutch ghost stories often tell of the Devil's presence in Stony Clove, a pass through the Devil's Path Range. Today, Stony Clove is better known as New York State Route 214, connecting the modern-day towns of Phoenicia and Hunter. The pass may be paved over, but the boulder known as the Devil's Tombstone remains. Almost 7 feet high and 5 feet across, the impressive monolith can be found at the southern end of the humble campground that bears its name. Presumably, it was deposited there by glacial activity or a landslide. No one knows for sure.

Surrounded by the Indian Head Wilderness, Devil's Tombstone is a secluded, primitive campground, only 4 miles from town, but seemingly far removed from civilization. It is one of the oldest collections of sites in the state, and NY 214 is the main reminder of the modern world. The road runs through the middle of the campground, dividing it into two sections. During the day, cars can be both seen and heard from most sites. Once

the sun sets, traffic reduces to a trickle, and it is unlikely you will even remember the road is there.

Upon arrival, be prepared to spend a little time checking in. Crowds are scarce and you probably won't be waiting in any lines, but the campground office is powered by a generator, which hardly provides enough energy to run the computer and printer at the same time. The ranger may treat you to tales of woebegone campers ignorant of how to pitch a tent, let alone start a fire, as he plugs your information into the database by the light of gas lamps.

They call Devil's Tombstone primitive camping, but the primary difference between this and other campgrounds in the region is the lack of running water in the comfort stations and the carry-out policy for all trash. The pit toilets are well maintained, and the comfort stations are sometimes even decorated with garlands of silk flowers. Potable-water spigots are well distributed throughout the campground. Supplies and groceries can be obtained in Hunter, a popular resort town only a few miles to the north. Campers in desperate need of a hot shower or a dip in a cold lake can drive a few miles east to Tannersville and use their Devil's Tombstone registration to gain free access to the facilities at North–South Lake (profiled later in this chapter).

:: Ratings

BEAUTY: ★ ★ ★
PRIVACY: ★ ★ ★
QUIET: ★ ★ ★ ★
CLEANLINESS: ★ ★ ★ ★
SECURITY: ★ ★
SPACIOUSNESS: ★ ★ ★

:: Key Information

ADDRESS: NY 214, P.O. Box 6,
Hunter, NY 12442

OPERATED BY: New York State Department of Environmental Conservation

CONTACT: 845-688-7160; www.dec.ny
.gov/outdoor/24462.html

OPEN: Mid-May–early October

SITES: 24

SITE AMENITIES: Picnic table and
fire ring

ASSIGNMENT: Choose from available
sites or reservations

REGISTRATION: On arrival

FACILITIES: Water, pit toilets, pay phone

PARKING: At site, maximum 2 vehicles

FEE: $16/night

ELEVATION: 1,902'

RESTRICTIONS:

■ Pets: Dogs on leash with proof of
currently valid rabies vaccination

■ Fires: In fire rings only

■ Alcohol: At site

■ Vehicles: Up to 30'

■ Other: Quiet hours 10 p.m.–7 a.m.; no
swimming or boating; carry out all trash

■ Reservations: 2-night stay required

The sites themselves are ample enough, and unless you're visiting on a holiday, it's rare to find the campground at capacity. On weekdays, only four or five sites at most may be filled. Personally, we found sites 3 and 4 on the eastern half of the campground the most desirable for their privacy. Some people prefer the western end, however, because it borders on Stony Clove Creek. Whether the creek is actually flowing when you visit is another story. Fed by the overflow of nearby Notch Lake, it will often run dry when rain hasn't made a recent visit. Partly because of the lack of facilities and possibly due to the challenging nature of the nearby hiking, the campground attracts fewer families and many more backpackers and young couples.

The satanic nomenclature is still appropriate today, as this is the jumping-off point for one of the most grueling hikes in the Catskills: the steep, rugged Devil's Path Trail. Just past the north end of the campground is a small parking lot bordering Notch Lake. At this point, the Devil's Path Trail bisects the road, leading west to

limited views, including a fire tower. To the east is the Plateau Hike, one of the most popular choices for day visitors because it provides gorgeous views of so many mountains that it is hard to tell where one ends and the next begins. The Plateau Hike takes about two hours round-trip, but this is hardly an afternoon ramble. The stony trail rises 1,700 feet in only 1.5 miles, ascending through dense forest. From the top, there are views of Hunter Mountain across Stony Clove and Slide Mountain to the south. The trail then loops around, offering views of Roundtop and Kaaterskill High Peak to the east. The Hudson Valley—and even Stratton and Mount Snow in Vermont—can be seen on clear days. Following the trail east will test even the most seasoned backpackers, but will reward with an authentic experience of the Indian Head Wilderness.

It would be difficult to overestimate the importance of this wild region. The Tombstone itself expresses this quite clearly. It holds a plaque from 1985 commemorating the 100th anniversary of the

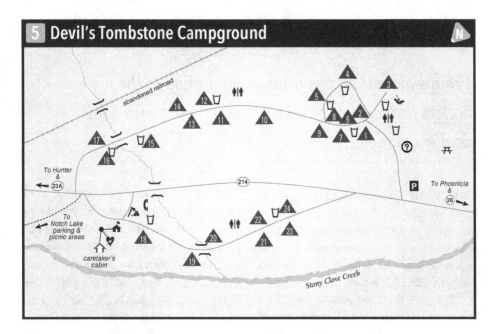

creation of the New York Forest Preserve, ending with these words: "The surrounding mountains, streams and woodlands remain a legacy from the past protected by the constitution of New York State. They represent a heritage for future generations."

:: Getting There

From I-87 (New York State Thruway), take Exit 19, Kingston, to NY 28 West. Follow NY 28 to the town of Phoenicia. In Phoenicia, follow the signs for NY 214. Drive 9 miles; the campground entrance is on the left.

GPS COORDINATES   N42° 09.400'   W74° 12.300'

6

Little Pond

Perhaps more than any other campground in the region, it offers the solitude of wilderness camping with a full catalog of amenities.

Little Pond Campground sits on the western edge of the Catskill Forest Preserve, just south of the Delaware River. Perhaps more than any other campground in the region, it offers the solitude of wilderness camping with a full catalog of amenities.

Don't let the word *pond* (or *little,* for that matter) fool you. In New York's Catskill and Adirondack Mountains, many bodies of water are dubbed ponds, but in different settings most would qualify as lakes. At 13 acres, Little Pond may not hold a candle to one of the Great Lakes, but it is hardly a puddle. Forested on all sides, it is a quiet spot to fish, swim, or paddle around in a small boat (no motorboats are allowed). And with a campground tucked along the southern shores, Little Pond makes for an excellent weekend getaway.

What struck us most about Little Pond Campground when we first entered was how lush the surroundings were. They bring to mind the Great Smoky Mountains in June.

:: Ratings

BEAUTY: ★ ★ ★ ★
PRIVACY: ★ ★ ★ ★
QUIET: ★ ★ ★ ★
CLEANLINESS: ★ ★ ★
SECURITY: ★ ★ ★
SPACIOUSNESS: ★ ★ ★ ★

The area is thin on population, but thick with wildlife. Upon registering, visitors are asked to read and sign a "Bear Warning and Guidelines Notification," outlining precautions to take when camping in the vicinity of black bears. New York has a population of approximately 7,000 black bears, and the region around Little Pond is indeed bear country. Although sightings are rare, for your own (as well as the bears') safety, you should take the guidelines seriously. It is easy to forget how dangerous bears can be. As one local ranger told us, "If you feed the chipmunks, you eventually feed the bears." The main camping area is divided into two sections, separated by a stream and a small pool of muddy water, which is perhaps more befitting of the campground's name. The loops are wooded, with tall trees rising from the red dirt. Rolling hills increase the sense of privacy. Each campsite features a fire ring, a picnic table, and a nice, flat place for a tent. Sites 1–21 are less hilly, a little more open, and farther from Little Pond. Sites 7, 8, 61, and 62 have views of the stream and the muddy pool. Some of the more popular sites are 25, 26, 35, 36, and 37, coveted for their proximity to Little Pond.

In addition to the main camping area, eight remote (that is, walk-in) sites are scattered along the north end of Little Pond. Campers staying at these sites can park at

:: Key Information

ADDRESS: 549 Little Pond State Campground Rd., Andes, NY 13731

OPERATED BY: New York State Department of Environmental Conservation

CONTACT: 845-439-5480; www.dec.ny .gov/outdoor/24478.html

OPEN: Mid-May–mid-October

SITES: 75 (including 8 walk-in sites)

SITE AMENITIES: Picnic table and fire ring

ASSIGNMENT: Choose from available sites or reservations

REGISTRATION: On arrival

FACILITIES: Water, pit and flush toilets, hot showers

PARKING: At site, maximum 2 vehicles or designated lot for walk-in sites

FEE: $22/night

ELEVATION: 1,657'

RESTRICTIONS:

■ **Pets:** Dogs on leash with proof of currently valid rabies vaccination

■ **Fires:** In fire rings only

■ **Alcohol:** At site

■ **Vehicles:** No maximum length

■ **Other:** Quiet hours 10 p.m.–7 a.m.; no motorized boats in Little Pond

■ **Reservations:** 2-night stay required

a lot next to the pond's boat ramp. A gravel nature trail with sturdy wooden bridges across streams starts at the lot and passes by an old stone fireplace before reaching the first site about 100 yards along. The sites are designated from 68 to 75, each with its own pit toilet and a view of the water. Site 71 is the most removed from the trail and closest to water. Site 73 offers excellent views. You may want to forgo site 72. Jutted up against the trail and small, it's the least-appealing option. Follow the trail past site 75 and skirt the edge of the pond until you reach the day-use area. Known as the Loop Trail, this short path is enjoyed by many families during the day, but when the sun goes down, the walk-in sites are quiet and private—a treat for tent campers.

Fishing is popular here, whether from the grassy banks, off the fishing pier, or over the edge of a boat. Canoes, kayaks, and rowboats are all available to rent, either by the hour or the day. Just down the road, fly fishers try their luck on the Beaverkill and the East Branch of the Delaware River. The largest bodies of water in the Catskills are a series of reservoirs that supply New York City. The nearby Pepacton Reservoir is full of large trout and bass, but permits obtained from New York City are needed to fish it.

Even if you're not a boater or an angler, you might enjoy the swimming beach and picnic area. In the summer, the campground offers a junior naturalist program for kids of all ages. Stock up on supplies at the Turnwood General Store less than a mile from the campground entrance. And if the nature trail is too short a jaunt for your tastes, you can set out from the day-use area and explore the base of Touchmenot Mountain and trails that continue on for miles to the east and west. Chances are, you will simply choose to stay at your campsite and enjoy the quiet surroundings.

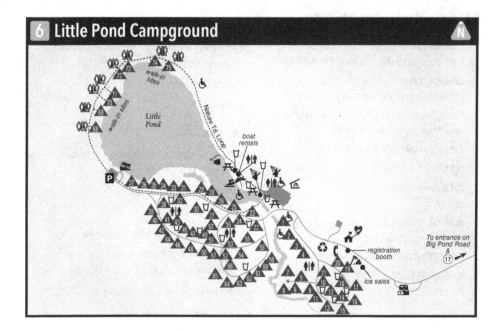

:: Getting There

From NY 17, take Exit 96, Livingston Manor, to Old Route 17. Follow Old Route 17 for 1 mile and turn right onto CR 151/Beaverkill Road. Follow CR 151 through the town of Lew Beach. After about 10 miles, make a left on Big Pond Road. Drive about 200 yards to the campground entrance, on the left.

GPS COORDINATES   N42° 02.133'   W74° 43.650'

7

Mills-Norrie State Park

This is where history and nature meet.

Ogden Mills and Ruth Livingston Mills Memorial State Park borders and shares a campground with Margaret Lewis Norrie State Park. The campground is technically located in Margaret Lewis Norrie, but understandably, its name was shortened to Mills-Norrie. Both parks are on the banks of the Hudson, and this is the state-park campground that's closest to the river. The Norrie Marina, which consists of a large boat launch and 145 rental slips, serves the campground and makes getting onto the water a snap.

We are unhappy to report that the campground is not directly on the water. It is perched upon a densely wooded hill, and the trees are too thick and the topography too sloped to afford river views. Unless you reserve one of the parks' 10 rental cabins, you will not be greeted by New York's most famous river when you wake. This is a blessing in some ways. Water views bring the unrelenting hordes, and Mills-Norrie is thankfully far from crowded.

Another welcome surprise at Mills-Norrie is its lack of RVs. There were none when we visited, and only a handful of pop-ups. RVs are certainly allowed and a few will make an appearance, but the sites themselves are small and somewhat crowded—a shame as far as privacy is concerned, but an obvious deterrent to noisy behemoths. The short, rough, intersecting roads may also help keep some trailers away.

The sites are arranged in a single loop, and as with many other campgrounds, the nicest spaces are located on the outer edge. Sites 48 and 49 are among the most private. Site 44, along the western edge, is not a bad option, but it's a bit exposed. The most coveted site would have to be 10. In the northwest corner, it is isolated, and if you walk a few paces and strain your eyes a bit, you might actually see the Hudson. In general, the campground fills up only on holiday weekends, so you can either reserve a site along the edge or simply show up and see which one strikes your fancy.

What brings most people to the campground is the chance to get their boat onto the Hudson River (there is no swimming within the park). While you can't launch your boat from your site, you are allowed to store it there, so long as it fits. Many locals rent seasonal slips at the bustling Norrie Marina, which is just down the road but well separated from the campground. Campers use the marina to launch small vessels, including plenty of kayaks, and the marina's parking lot usually accommodates their cars and trailers. An environmental center, just south of the lot at the edge of the park boundary, offers programs here on Saturdays in the summer. It is also a good place to

:: Ratings

BEAUTY: ★ ★
PRIVACY: ★ ★
QUIET: ★ ★ ★
CLEANLINESS: ★ ★
SECURITY: ★ ★
SPACIOUSNESS: ★ ★

:: Key Information

ADDRESS: 9 Old Post Rd., P.O. Box 308, Staatsburg, NY 12580	**PARKING:** At site, maximum 2 vehicles
OPERATED BY: New York State Office of Parks, Recreation and Historic Preservation	**FEE:** $15/night (plus $4/night on Fridays, Saturdays, and holidays)
	ELEVATION: 30'
CONTACT: 845-889-4646; nysparks .com/parks/171/details.aspx	**RESTRICTIONS:**
OPEN: Mid-May–late October	▥ **Pets:** Household pets caged or on leash; proof of currently valid rabies vaccination for dogs; maximum 2 pets per site
SITES: 46	
SITE AMENITIES: Picnic table and fire ring	
ASSIGNMENT: Choose from available sites or reservations	▥ **Fires:** In fire rings only
	▥ **Alcohol:** At site
REGISTRATION: On arrival	▥ **Vehicles:** Up to 40'
FACILITIES: Water, flush toilets, hot showers	▥ **Other:** Quiet hours 10 p.m.–7 a.m.
	▥ **Reservations:** 2-night stay required unless booked within 3 days of arrival

set off on some of the parks' trails and into almost 1,000 acres of forests and fields.

For gorgeous vistas of the Hudson, grab the trail map from the environmental center and take a hike north on the White Trail, which visits the campground and follows along bluffs, high above the water. The Horse Trail and the Mills Historic Trail make their way through the center of the parks, the latter ending at Mills Mansion (a.k.a. Staatsburgh State Historic Site), a pillared 79-room Beaux Arts estate donated by the Mills family to the state in 1938. Tours are available Wednesdays–Sundays during camping season. For a short, looping stroll, try the Yellow Trail, which can be accessed from a parking lot near the campground. Three other color-blazed trails—Blue, Red, and Green—follow old dirt roads, and double as cross-country ski paths in the winter.

Mills-Norrie is truly at the heart of the historic Hudson Valley, where industrialists and influential figures maintained extravagant homes. Aside from Mills Mansion,

many other important buildings are minutes away. Five miles south is the town of Hyde Park, home to the Vanderbilt Mansion, Franklin Delano Roosevelt's Springwood and Presidential Library, and Eleanor Roosevelt's cottage, Val-Kill. Hop over the Mid-Hudson Bridge and drive about 40 minutes to visit Mohonk Mountain House, an elegant and gigantic castle that is one of the country's most famous hotels. You won't have to book a room, but you will have to pay an entrance fee to explore the estate's impeccable gardens and miles of hiking trails.

Admittedly, the campground at Mills-Norrie is not the most inspired. It could use some more maintenance (though the comfort stations were clean and new when we visited), and security is not its strong point. It is, however, in a wonderful location, close to the wide shores of the Hudson. More than anywhere else in the state, this is where history and nature meet. Whether by boat, by foot, or by car, you can easily access it all from Mills-Norrie.

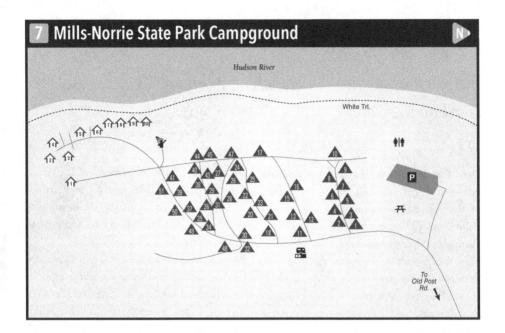

7 Mills-Norrie State Park Campground

:: Getting There

From I-87 (New York State Thruway), take Exit 19, Kingston. Follow NY 199 East over the Kingston–Rhinecliff Bridge to US 9G South. Follow US 9G South 1.5 miles, then turn right on US 9 South. Follow US 9 South 5 miles to the village of Staatsburg, and turn right on Old Post Road. The park entrance is on the right.

GPS COORDINATES   N41° 50.417'   W73° 55.833'

8

Mongaup Pond

Gas engines are prohibited here, making for a calm, leisurely spirit on the water.

The Catskill Fish Hatchery, a rather unassuming complex but an important part of the regional economy, lies less than 3 miles from the entrance of Mongaup Pond Campground. It provides fish to local waterways that attract a large percentage of the visitors to the western edge of the Catskill Forest Preserve. Mongaup Creek, Willowemoc Stream, and the Delaware River are favorites of those who can tie a good fly. And boat-bound anglers make pilgrimages to Long Pond, Frick Pond, Quick Lake, Hodge Pond, Waneta Lake, and especially Mongaup Pond, home to chain pickerel, golden shiner pumpkinseed, yellow bullhead, yellow perch, smallmouth bass, and white sucker.

They call it a pond, but Mongaup is a lake by most standards, and at 120 acres, it is actually the largest body of water in the Catskills outside of the reservoirs that serve New York City. Gas engines are prohibited, making for a calm, leisurely spirit on the water. The car-top boat launch next to the fishing pier sees a lot of traffic, and rowboats and canoes are plentiful (and available

:: Ratings

BEAUTY: ★ ★ ★
PRIVACY: ★ ★ ★
QUIET: ★ ★ ★ ★
CLEANLINESS: ★ ★ ★ ★
SECURITY: ★ ★ ★ ★
SPACIOUSNESS: ★ ★ ★ ★ ★

for rent). At the southern end of the pond, a picnic area, a large, sandy beach, and a roped-off section of water for swimming draw some day-use visitors in addition to most campers.

During the summer, organized environmental and recreational activities for both children and adults are posted in the *Wilderness Times*, a newsletter available at the ranger station. The campground also participates in the state-run Junior Naturalist Program. Children between the ages of 5 and 12 can fill out a wildlife journal to earn a colorful patch. A recent year's patch depicted a black bear, an animal that's actually somewhat common in surrounding Sullivan County. The staff asks campers registering to sign a bear-notification form and warns them to take precautions, including not sleeping in clothes worn while cooking.

Isolation reigns at Mongaup, and there is no private development on the lake—just the seven loops of sites, all suitable for tents or RVs. The sections are so well spaced that it is easy to forget there are more than 160 sites. Each is standard-issue, but a few small touches in the campground really stand out. The faux stone on fireplaces and bright flowers planted near the showers and boat ramp were evidence of a well-maintained facility when we visited. The occasional pop-up will stop over for a visit, but even fewer RVs pass through the gates. Families in tents are definitely the majority here. The staff is very

:: Key Information

ADDRESS: 231 Mongaup Pond Rd., Livingston Manor, NY 12758

OPERATED BY: New York State Department of Environmental Conservation

CONTACT: 845-439-4233; www.dec.ny .gov/outdoor/24484.html

OPEN: Mid-May–mid-October

SITES: 163

SITE AMENITIES: Picnic table and fire ring

ASSIGNMENT: Choose from available sites or reservations

REGISTRATION: On arrival

FACILITIES: Water, flush toilets, hot showers, pay phone

PARKING: At site, maximum 2 vehicles

FEE: $22/night

ELEVATION: 2,146'

RESTRICTIONS:

◼ **Pets:** Dogs on leash with proof of currently valid rabies vaccination

◼ **Fires:** In fire rings only

◼ **Alcohol:** At site

◼ **Vehicles:** Up to 30'

◼ **Other:** Quiet hours 10 p.m.–7 a.m.; no motorboats except for electric motors with less than 25 pounds of thrust

◼ **Reservations:** 2-night stay required

conscious of human impact on the campground and encourages campers to stay in the middle of their sites to prevent them from expanding over time.

Loops A, B, and C are spread out along the southeast section of the pond, just past the registration booth. In general, the interior sections of the loops provide less privacy but are closer to the comfort stations. Loops A and B are not on the lake and include some of the more crowded sites, such as 32–36, 53, 55, and 67–69. Behind sites 42, 44, and 46, a large field calls out for a game of ball. Loop C has a smattering of sites with water views, but the more-spacious Loops D, E, F, and G offer better options for those seeking memorable views. Loops D and E contain the largest sites available, sitting beneath the shade of older hardwoods. On Loops F and G, denser, smaller trees and shrubs envelop the sites, and campers are guaranteed a little more privacy. The waterfront sites at Loop F are some of the most popular, most notably 122–124, 126–130, and 132–136. Loop G, the

farthest from both the registration booth and day-use area, is also not too shabby. For a quieter waterfront sojourn, 139–144 are the best options.

The twisting coastline of Mongaup Pond allows for a total of 50 sites with water views. But few are directly at the water's edge. That's not such a bad thing, for it increases the sense of seclusion when looking out over the pond. But at night, it's certainly pleasant to see the twinkling lights of campfires across the water.

Supplies are easy to come by, as the Woodman and Happy Trails traveling stores, in the form of pickup trucks or small vans, circle the loops at least once every evening. In addition to helping keep you or your food warm, the Woodman sells ice to keep your drinks and perishables cool. Happy Trails provides everything campers could need, ranging from food (ice cream, chips, soda) to practical (duct tape, batteries, bug spray) and purely fun items (magic-grow capsules, glow sticks, hula hoops).

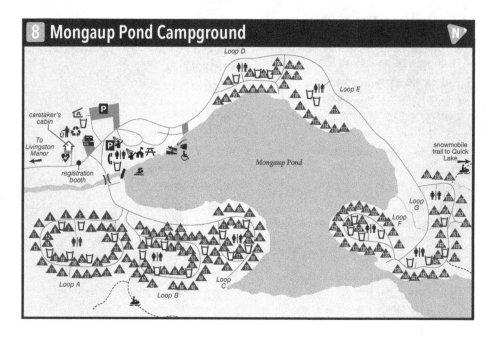

For those seeking activities beyond their campsites, there are miles of multi-use trails nearby. A popular short hike, the 3.5-mile Waterfall Loop, passes a cascade of water and the site of an old sawmill. Hikers will find trails to Long Pond and Mongaup Mountain leaving directly from the campground. The Frick Pond trailhead, offering longer trails to the northwest, has its own parking lot, located down a short road to the west just before the campground entrance.

Whether you seek a destination for boating, swimming, hiking, or just a nice campfire, Mongaup Pond is sure to offer something for all tent campers. Be sure to pack that tackle box, though. About 58 tons of brown trout are produced at the hatchery every year and released locally. You're bound to pull up a pound or two in nearby waters.

:: Getting There

From NY 17, take Exit 96, Livingston Manor, to CR 81/82 and follow it 6 miles. In the village of Debruce, turn left on Mongaup Road/Fish Hatchery Road and follow it 3 miles to the campground entrance, straight ahead.

GPS COORDINATES   N41° 57.383'   W74° 41.483'

9

North–South Lake

For a community-camping experience, North–South Lake is fantastic during the summer.

The largest and most popular campground in the Catskills, North–South Lake hardly qualifies as an undiscovered gem. Its popularity, however, is well deserved and should not discourage the camper looking for excellent hiking and recreation opportunities. Easily accessible from the New York State Thruway and a stone's throw from the ski-resort town of Hunter, North–South Lake has served as an ideal jumping-off point for exploring the northeastern Catskills for many years.

Even those who have never visited the area may recognize the scenery from the work of the Hudson River School of early American painters. Nearby Kaaterskill Falls, the highest falls in the state, is depicted in Thomas Cole's *Falls of the Kaaterskill,* and North–South Lake served as inspiration to Jasper Francis Cropsey and his 1850 painting *Catskill Creek.*

The name North–South Lake is, of course, a curious one. The lake is currently a single entity, but for most of its history an earthen dam in a narrow isthmus separated it into two bodies of water. In 1929, the state established a 10-site campground on North Lake. Yet it was not until 1984, when the state purchased South Lake from a private owner, that the dam was removed and North–South Lake in its present form was born. People still refer to North Lake and South Lake for the sake of clarity.

While the number of campsites in the campground has blossomed to 219 over the years, the sites are still restricted to the shores and surrounding forest of North Lake. South Lake is home to a parking lot, a beach, and a rentable picnic pavilion, but is open for day use only. North Lake also includes a day-use area, with a beach, picnic tables, fireplaces, charcoal grills, and its own pavilion. Both beaches are pleasant and well maintained and allow swimming from Memorial Day to Labor Day, but only when lifeguards are on duty.

The campground is separated into seven one-way loops, four of which border the shores of the lake. Be aware that not all loops may be open early and late in the season, and each loop will offer a slightly different experience depending on its size and location. Loops 2, 4, and 7 do not have lakefront sites but tend to be quieter, with Loop 7 being the most private. The largest is Loop 3, which offers a limited number of handicap-accessible sites. Loop 5 includes some of the best sites in the campground, particularly 145–148, which are footsteps from the water's edge.

:: Ratings

BEAUTY: ★ ★ ★ ★
PRIVACY: ★ ★ ★
QUIET: ★ ★ ★
CLEANLINESS: ★ ★ ★ ★
SECURITY: ★ ★ ★ ★
SPACIOUSNESS: ★ ★ ★ ★

:: Key Information

ADDRESS: CR 18, P.O. Box 347, Haines Falls, NY 12436

OPERATED BY: New York State Department of Environmental Conservation

CONTACT: 518-589-5058; www.dec.ny.gov/outdoor/24487.html

OPEN: Early May–late October

SITES: 219

SITE AMENITIES: Picnic table and fire ring

ASSIGNMENT: Choose from available sites or reservations

REGISTRATION: On arrival or by reservation

FACILITIES: Water, flush toilets, showers

PARKING: At site, maximum 2 vehicles

FEE: $22/night

ELEVATION: 2,250'

RESTRICTIONS:

- **Pets:** Dogs on leash with proof of currently valid rabies vaccination
- **Fires:** In fire rings only
- **Alcohol:** At site
- **Vehicles:** Pop-up campers allowed
- **Other:** Quiet hours 10 p.m.–7 a.m.
- **Reservations:** 2-night stay required

Each loop is equipped with at least one comfort station with flush toilets and multiple water sources. Hot showers are always a short walk away. The well-maintained and exceptionally clean facilities are worth the occasional inconvenience caused by construction and maintenance projects. At the exit of the campground are a trailer dump station and a trash and recycling center, making disposal of waste an easy task.

Unsurprisingly, lakefront sites tend to be the most popular, but all sites are heavily wooded, offering adequate privacy. Reservations are recommended at all times and necessary during summer weekends and holidays, with a two-night minimum stay required. Book early to obtain a lakefront site: it is well worth the effort. Sites are designated for tents and trailers only, with a pull-through parking area (two vehicles and two tents maximum), picnic table, and fire ring. There are no full-service sites in the campground, so RVs are few and far between. Rangers regularly patrol the grounds and quiet hours are strictly enforced from 10 p.m. to 7 a.m.

The campground's popularity allows for a wide variety of organized activities. From late June to Labor Day, the posted *Wilderness Times* includes times and information on all group activities, from nature hikes to crafts, games, and live entertainment.

Fishing is permitted, and anglers can find a number of species in the lake, including brown bullhead, largemouth bass, chain pickerel, and pumpkinseed. No motorboats are allowed, but rental rowboats, canoes, kayaks, and paddleboats are available. A paved boat ramp can be accessed at the North Lake day-use area.

More than any other campground in the region, North–South Lake offers the outdoors enthusiast a variety of hiking trails, including the well-traveled Escarpment Trail, Rock Shelter Trail, Mary's Glen Trail, and Schutt Road Trail. Artists' Rock lies about a half-mile from the campground along the Escarpment Trail and is just one of many spots for picturesque views. Farther along the Escarpment Trail is North Point, where even the hardiest day hikers usually decide to turn around. Alligator

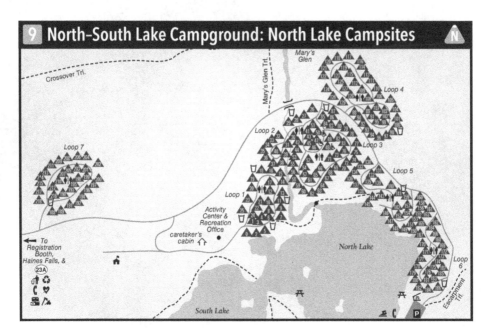

Rock (featuring "teeth" added by visitors over the years) is a favorite spot for families with small children. The now-vacant sites of the once-lavish 19th-century Kaaterskill Hotel and Catskill Mountain House are also easy to reach, and serve as a reminder of the area's rich history as a 200-year-old vacation destination.

For a community camping experience, North–South Lake is fantastic during the summer. But for a quieter visit, consider the spring or fall (when the foliage is at its peak).

:: Getting There

From I-87 (New York State Thruway), take NY 32 North 6 miles to NY 32A. Follow NY 32A briefly to NY 23A West. In Haines Falls, turn right on CR 18. Drive 2 miles to the campground.

GPS COORDINATES   N42° 11.867'   W74° 04.133'

10

Peekamoose

It's all free of charge on a first-come, first-serve basis, and the sites are large, flat, shady, and private.

At the southern end of the Catskills, in the Sundown Wild Forest, lies the Peekamoose Valley, where three 2,000-foot peaks—Samson, Van Wyck, and Peekamoose Mountains—funnel water into Rondout Creek through a series of picturesque waterfalls. In the midst of all of this is a campground that, while administered by the state Department of Environmental Conservation (DEC), is decidedly different from any of the Catskills' other offerings. If you're looking for a place to pitch your tent that's somewhere between backcountry camping and primitive but is an established property such as Devil's Tombstone (see page 25), then you'll find this is your sweet spot (or 25 sweet spots, to be more exact).

The campground is stretched out over a mile and is made up of three separate fields, each containing six to nine walk-in sites. (There's also a trailer field that requires permits; contact the DEC for more information on that area.) There's no running water, no trash pickup, no picnic tables, and only seasonal porta-potties at the parking lots. But it's all free of charge on a first-come,

first-serve basis, and the sites are large, flat, shady, and private. From nearly every corner of the campground, you can hear the sound of trickling Rondout Creek.

Each site is limited to nine people and three tents. Part of the fun is exploring the winding paths to discover the best available spot for you. Be careful to select a site with a designated camping sign, as the DEC occasionally rotates locations to spread out the impact of campers. Admittedly, some of the former sites can be very tempting. And don't let the name "field" fool you; only a few sites are actually in fields. Most are nicely wooded options with ample vegetation.

As you approach from the northeast along Peekamoose Road/CR 42, the first area after the trailer field is the Upper Field with its two parking lots. Closest to the eastern lot, sites 1 and 2 sit across from the trailer field along a dry creek bed (or at least it's been dry when we have visited). Sites 3 and 5 are closer to the road, but are nicely situated among spruce trees on the opposite side of the field's well-worn main trail. Numbers 4 and 8 are even closer to the trail, while 6 and 7 are tucked away on little spurs near the western parking lot.

Farther along Peekamoose Road, toward Sundown, the Middle Field features six sites and one small parking lot. While sites 1 and 2 (set off to the right of the lot) are both close to the creek, they are also somewhat close to the road. Still, they're a better choice than site 3, which is within spitting distance

:: Ratings

BEAUTY: ★ ★ ★ ★
PRIVACY: ★ ★ ★
QUIET: ★ ★
CLEANLINESS: ★ ★
SECURITY: ★
SPACIOUSNESS: ★ ★ ★ ★

:: Key Information

ADDRESS: CR 42, Denning, NY 12725	**FEE:** Free
OPERATED BY: New York State Department of Environmental Conservation	**ELEVATION:** 1,096'
CONTACT: 845-240-6788; www.dec.ny.gov/lands/75346.html	**RESTRICTIONS:**
OPEN: Year-round	■ **Pets:** Dogs on leash with proof of currently valid rabies vaccination
SITES: About 25	■ **Fires:** In fire rings only
SITE AMENITIES: Fire ring	■ **Alcohol:** At site
ASSIGNMENT: Choose from available sites; no reservations	■ **Vehicles:** None permitted; all sites are walk-in
REGISTRATION: Not required	■ **Other:** Quiet hours 10 p.m.–7 a.m. (not enforced)
FACILITIES: Portable toilets June–September	■ **Reservations:** None taken, but call ahead if you're planning to stay more than 3 nights.
PARKING: At designated lots	

of the parking lot. We prefer sites 4 and 5 for their privacy and their soft, sandy perches next to the creek (and a nice little swimming hole), along with site 6 for its grassy seclusion near an open field. As in other parts of the campground, small, dry creek beds (some used as default trails) crisscross near most of the sites, so be wary during periods of heavy rain.

The Lower Field, not much farther down the road, houses nine sites. The sites are nicely spread and, thanks to their distance from the large parking lot and their location across an old bridge, they tend to be the quietest choices. From the lot, walk down a hill, cross the bridge to the information kiosk, and you will find sites 1–6 to the right and sites 7–9 to the left. For the most privacy, check out site 1. About a quarter-mile removed from the rest of the sites past an old stone wall, it's remote and woodsy enough for the greatest of recluses. Site 3 is not far from the edge of the creek. Numbers 2, 4, 5 (the largest), and 6 are all scattered along the edge of a tall grass field bordering

a steep hill thick with fir trees that cast shade upon the sites. Number 7 sits just past the information kiosk, while 8 and 9 (always good choices) are closer to the creek and are often home to some interesting camper-created art made with stones worn smooth by the water.

Because there are no reservations, you could show up and find the campground already full. On the plus side, impromptu getaways can be rewarded with free streamside campsites and absolutely no paperwork. Still, summer weekends fill up fast, so don't arrive after dark on a Friday evening and expect luck to be on your side. Local DEC rangers do occasionally patrol, but rules, especially quiet hours, are treated differently by all. Be wary of rowdy parties, especially on holiday weekends. Previous tenants may leave presents for you, ranging from trash bags to well-stacked stone cairns. Just because there's no staff on-site, be sure to leave Peekamoose as you would like to find it.

In the surrounding Peekamoose Valley, you'll find a stunning swimming hole,

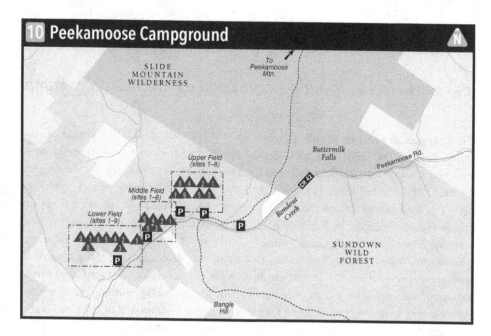

10 Peekamoose Campground

lots of accessible waterfalls, and a variety of hiking options. Across the road from the upper field's eastern lot, a large boulder marks the trailhead to Bangle Hill and Vernooy Kill Falls, and just east along Peekamoose Road is the Peekamoose–Table Trail, a strenuous route that rewards the industrious hiker with great views. For an easier route to views, drive to the nearby town of Denning for a 1.2-mile hike to Red Hill Fire Tower. After all that climbing and sweating, you'll want to cool off with a trip to the famous Blue Hole, a legendary swimming hole just 2 miles east along Peekamoose Road. It's chilly even in the peak of summer, but don't let that stop you from taking a memorable leap into the crystal-clear water.

:: Getting There

From I-87 (New York State Thruway), take Exit 19, New York 28/Kingston/Rhinecliff Bridge. At the traffic circle, take the first exit and follow NY 28 West 16 miles. Take a slight left onto NY 28A/New York City Road for 3 miles. Make a slight right onto CR 42 West/West Shokan-Peekamoose-Sundown Road, and drive 11 miles to the Upper Field entrance, on the right.

GPS COORDINATES   N41° 54.567'   W74° 27.217'

11

Taconic State Park: Copake Falls Area

It's easy to feel as if you've come upon a family summer camp.

On the eastern edge of the Hudson Valley, hugging the borders of Massachusetts and Connecticut, Taconic State Park stretches for nearly 15 miles along a thin stretch of land in the Taconic Mountains, broken only occasionally by privately held property. There are two separate campgrounds in Taconic State Park. On its southern end is the Rudd Pond Area, which consists of a narrow lake and an even narrower clearing with compact camping sites. The campground's open field seems more like an afterthought, and in stark contrast to the nicely shaded campground found at the Copake Falls Area on the park's northern end. For exploring the region, Copake Falls is the clear choice among places to pitch a tent.

As you enter, it's easy to feel as if you've come upon a family summer camp. Groups of cyclists crisscross the road in front of the Depot Deli, a popular lunch destination and store, which is directly across from the campground entrance. Just through the park gates on the left side of the road is a shallow pond that swarms with small children on hot summer days. Connected to this wading pool is what appears to be a small lake. It is actually a former mining pit filled with water. Known (appropriately enough) as Ore Pit Pond, it is spring-fed and reaches depths of 40 feet. Although there is no beach, a sturdy dock skirts the edge of the water. Both the wading pool and Ore Pit Pond open for weekend swimming on Memorial Day, then expand to weekday use at the end of June, and finally close on Labor Day. From 11 a.m. to 7 p.m., swimming is allowed, and both locals and campers take advantage.

Farther along the road are the park's remaining day-use facilities, including picnic tables, grills, comfort stations, showers, and a baseball diamond—all situated for easy access from a large parking lot. A nature center, just north of the parking lot, provides programs on Saturdays and Sundays for all ages. Little more than a cabin, the center is filled with animal skulls, interesting geologic samples, leaves from the park's variety of trees, topographic maps, and a large tree-trunk cutaway, the rings of which present a time line of the park's history. Young naturalists will not be disappointed.

The campground itself is located at the end of the road to the east of the parking lot, nestled on a wooded slope. Towering hemlocks shade a collection of somewhat crowded sites in the center of the A Area. The campground was once even more congested, and in recent years the park has removed more than 15 sites. That may not seem obvious at first, but sites become more secluded in the B Area, located directly east

:: Ratings

BEAUTY: ★ ★ ★
PRIVACY: ★ ★
QUIET: ★ ★ ★
CLEANLINESS: ★ ★ ★
SECURITY: ★ ★ ★
SPACIOUSNESS: ★ ★ ★

:: Key Information

ADDRESS: NY 344, P.O. Box 100, Copake Falls, NY 12517

OPERATED BY: New York State Office of Parks, Recreation and Historic Preservation

CONTACT: 518-329-3993; nysparks .com/parks/83/details.aspx

OPEN: Early May–early December

SITES: 46 tent sites, 24 tent-platform sites, and 36 trailer sites

SITE AMENITIES: Picnic table and fire ring with grate

ASSIGNMENT: Choose from available sites or reservations

REGISTRATION: On arrival

FACILITIES: Water, pit and flush toilets, showers

PARKING: At site, maximum 2 vehicles

FEE: $15/night (plus $4/night on Fridays, Saturdays, and holidays)

ELEVATION: 786'

RESTRICTIONS:

■ **Pets:** Dogs in D Area only, on leash and with proof of currently valid rabies vaccination

■ **Fires:** In fire rings only

■ **Alcohol:** At site

■ **Vehicles:** Up to 30'

■ **Other:** Quiet hours 10 p.m.–7 a.m.

■ **Reservations:** 2-night stay required

and uphill along the campground road. B-64 is one of the better sites, a private and spacious spot that is often the first choice for tent campers. Platform sites are scattered throughout the A and B Areas, and are often necessary, as some parts of the campground are steeper than others.

Dogs are allowed, but only in the D Area, which consists exclusively of combination trailer–tent sites. There are no electric or water hookups in the campground, but RVs are directed to the C Area at the northwest corner of the campground. The park supervisor told us that they may convert some of the tent sites to trailer sites in the future, but there will still be plenty of sites exclusively for tent camping.

In addition to the land encompassed by Taconic State Park, many trails stretch into the Berkshire Mountains in Massachusetts, and visitors to Copake Falls can easily walk over the border and visit Bash Bish Falls and Mount Washington State Forest. Bash Bish

Falls is one of the most popular day hikes accessible from the campground, but campers can choose from more than 25 miles of hiking trails, ranging from easy to difficult.

Bike rentals are available just outside the campground entrance, where NY 344 is bisected by the Harlem Valley Rail Trail, a flat, paved path for walkers, runners, and cyclists. There are plans to develop the Harlem Valley Rail Trail so that it will one day stretch for 46 unbroken miles. Currently, some sections of the trail are not complete, but visitors can travel from one piece of the trail to the next along local roads through the rolling farmland. It is such a pleasure to drive on these roads, and exploring them at a slower pace on foot or bike makes for a lovely detour.

For people who do not find a few flaps of nylon to be adequate accommodations (surely not readers of this book), Copake Falls also has cabins. Iron ore was mined here for years, and the cabins are remnants of that

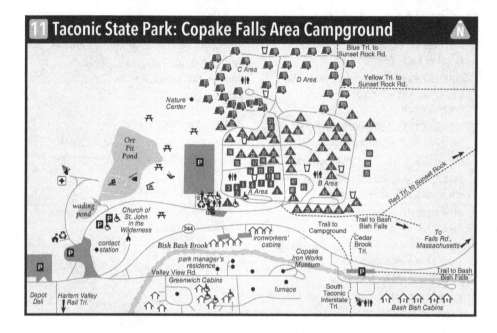

11 Taconic State Park: Copake Falls Area Campground

time. Restored and available to rent, they are a unique alternative to a motel. You can learn more about the industrial history of the park at the Copake Iron Works Museum, a short distance down the road from the cabins.

The annual Falcon Ridge Folk Festival brings many campers to the park for the dancing and performances in nearby Hillsdale. Beyond Hillsdale, the surrounding area of Columbia County has a number of family activities, but the area's parks definitely offer enough to keep visitors busy for a weekend getaway or even an entire week's vacation.

:: Getting There

From Taconic State Parkway, take the Claverack/Hillsdale exit. Follow NY 23 East 8 miles. In the village of Hillsdale, turn right on NY 22 South. Follow NY 22 South 4 miles. In the village of Copake Falls, turn left on NY 344 East. Follow NY 344 East 0.5 mile; the park entrance is on the left.

GPS COORDINATES N42° 07.250' W73° 31.167'

12

Woodland Valley

If you want to walk directly from your tent onto some of the most popular trails in the region, this is the campground for you.

When one speaks of hiking in the Catskill Park, it is hard not to mention Slide Mountain. At 4,190 feet, Slide is the highest peak in the Catskills and the crown jewel of the Slide Mountain Wilderness, which makes up 47,500 acres of the park. Great hiking abounds here, and since Woodland Valley Campground is centrally located, it services backpackers and families alike. Sure, the more spacious Kenneth Wilson Campground is only 13 miles away, and is a nice place to start your explorations of the central Catskills. But if you want to walk directly from your tent onto some of the most popular trails in the region, Woodland Valley is the campground for you.

As you enter the facilities, you'll come across the park ranger's office, a comfort station, the day-use parking area, and the Slide–Wittenberg Trailhead and the Woodland Valley–Denning Trailhead (which leads to the Giant Ledge–Slide Mountain Trail). These hikes, leading up both sides of the steep valley, are heavily trafficked, and the day-use area can fill up, with parking areas sometimes overflowing on very busy weekends. If you want to tackle Slide Mountain or other peaks, such as Wittenberg, Panther, Terrace, or Cornell, it's worth the few extra dollars to reserve a campsite at Woodland Valley, guaranteeing you both a parking spot and an early-morning start.

Featuring two strips of standard sites divided by Woodland Valley Road, the campground can seem a little cramped and close to traffic. But the road comes to a dead end just past the western edge of the campground, so you need not worry about any cars passing through and disturbing the quiet. The campground also lacks power hookups, and many of the sites do not have parking areas large enough to fit even a trailer, so tents are definitely in the majority.

Most of the sites are on the southern edge of Woodland Valley Road, bordering Woodland Valley Stream. Sites 1–15 are rather congested, so when making a reservation (recommended on weekends and holidays), choose sites in the 20s and 30s for their privacy. Site 25, sitting next to the rocky stream on a spur from the camp road, is among the most desired. On the opposite side of Woodland Valley Road are sites 50–69, which skirt the edge of cliffs and are

:: Ratings

BEAUTY: ★ ★ ★ ★
PRIVACY: ★ ★ ★
QUIET: ★ ★ ★
CLEANLINESS: ★ ★ ★
SECURITY: ★ ★ ★
SPACIOUSNESS: ★ ★ ★

:: Key Information

ADDRESS: 1319 Woodland Valley Rd., Phoenicia, NY 12464

OPERATED BY: New York State Department of Environmental Conservation

CONTACT: 845-688-7647; www.dec.ny.gov/outdoor/24501.html

OPEN: Mid-May–mid-October

SITES: 72

SITE AMENITIES: Picnic table and fire ring

ASSIGNMENT: Choose from available sites or reservations

REGISTRATION: On arrival

FACILITIES: Water, flush toilets, hot showers, pay phone

PARKING: At site, maximum 2 vehicles

FEE: $20/night

ELEVATION: 1,368'

RESTRICTIONS:

■ **Pets:** Dogs on leash with proof of currently valid rabies vaccination

■ **Fires:** In fire rings only

■ **Alcohol:** At site

■ **Vehicles:** Up to 30'

■ **Other:** Quiet hours 10 p.m.–7 a.m.

■ **Reservations:** 2-night stay required

farther from the crowd, but also farther from the pleasant sound of the water.

Woodland Valley Stream, a tributary of Esopus Creek, occasionally dries up, but when running, it offers fishing for three types of trout. The camp staff discourages swimming and wading, as no area in the campground is designated for such use, so use your best judgment if you decide to enter the water. Nearby Kenneth Wilson Campground has a lake offering a sandy beach and boat rentals. Use your camping receipt to gain free access to its facilities during the length of your stay at Woodland Valley.

Some campers bike the 6 miles into Phoenicia along the windy Woodland Valley Road. In this small resort town, you'll easily find camp supplies, antiques stores, restaurants, and gift shops. An interesting sight is the line that can form in the evening at the town's one pay phone: cell phone reception is especially poor in the valley. At the edge of town is a large RV park that draws the more motorized crowd.

Whether you're staying in a tent, an RV, or a bed-and-breakfast, you'll find a number of popular tourist activities in the area. Tubing in Esopus Creek is the perfect way to stay cool during hot summer days. Local outfitters will supply transportation, flotation, and safety gear. The Catskill Mountain Railroad offers scenic rides and a rail shuttle to transport tubers upstream. The historic rail route also provides a fall-foliage route for the many leaf-peepers who fill the park every October.

Still, hiking is what this area is known for. Even when going for only a short walk in the woods, be sure to consult the park ranger for information on local trails and conditions. Use common sense to avoid getting lost, and always carry some basic supplies, such as water, snacks, extra clothing, and first-aid supplies. Remember that conditions on mountaintops and at night can vary drastically from those on the valley floor and during the day. A topographic map is a great help to plan for the different elevations you may encounter on the trail.

Even if you don't take advantage of the many trails in the area, do take a moment to look at a topographical map. A meteor

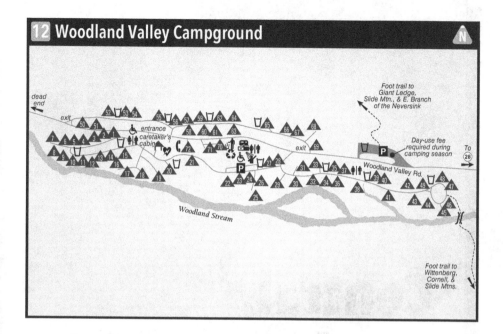

impact 350 million years ago left an outline of an almost-perfect circle around what is now Panther Mountain. This ring is nearly 7 miles in diameter and clearly marked by Esopus Creek and Woodland Valley Stream. What was once a sunken meteor site is now one of the highest mountains in the Catskills, overlooking thickly wooded land that offers some of the best hiking in New York.

:: Getting There

From I-87 (New York State Thruway), take Exit 19, Kingston, to NY 28 West. Follow NY 28 West 26 miles. In Phoenicia, just before a bridge and railroad tracks, turn left on Woodland Valley Road/High Street. Follow Woodland Valley Road/High Street 6 miles; the campground entrance is on the left.

GPS COORDINATES   N42° 02.133'   W74° 21.733'

Central, Leatherstocking, and Capital

13

Bowman Lake State Park

Keep an eye out for white-tailed deer, red foxes, woodchucks, beavers, and a wide variety of birds.

Bowman Lake State Park advertises itself as a "camper's paradise"—an exaggerated claim, perhaps, but not entirely inaccurate. It has nearly 200 campsites, including some designated for tents only, to go along with seven new camping cabins. Quaint signposts throughout the park have been constructed from rough-hewn wood and bespeak a commitment to providing a natural experience. Trees are thick, from maples and beech to cherry, pine, and dogwood. And ferns abound on the forest floor. It may not be located in the nearly boundless wilderness of the Adirondacks or Catskills, but it often seems that way.

Located about 30 miles north of Binghamton, Bowman Lake State Park opened in the 1960s. Since then, it has strived to provide campers from central New York with a more private alternative to Gilbert Lake, Oquagua Creek, Chenango Valley, and other state parks in the region. But it is not some tiny hideaway, where there is nothing to do but pitch a tent. At 653 acres, it is a smaller park, but its facilities are the size of many

larger parks. It has the proverbial beach and miles of trails to explore. Snicker if you like at the signs with raccoons on them that read, "I'm cute and I bite. And I may have rabies." But they're a good reminder that this is the wild—you will be sharing the park with animals, and you should respect any advice the experienced staff provides.

The campground is arranged in a series of overlapping loops, which can make for a confusing drive when trying to find your site. Yet it gives each site a unique vantage point. Sites 156–161 and 170–192 (plus wheelchair-accessible sites 193–195) have been established as tent-only. Sites 162–169 are no longer used and have therefore disappeared from the campground map. Be warned, though: just because a site is listed as tent-only, that doesn't mean it's a winner. There is little reason to reserve sites 156–161. They seem as if they've been tacked on, distributed along the edges of parking lots—not technically designated as overflow, but not technically appealing either.

Sites 170–195 occupy a small private loop on the southern edge of the campground, directly past the park office and near a shower building and a small playground. As much as we applaud the park for providing these tent-only sites, you'd probably do well to choose a site elsewhere, especially during the week or in the off-season, when RVs are not choking the campground roads: the multiuse sites tend to be larger

:: Ratings

BEAUTY: ★ ★ ★
PRIVACY: ★ ★ ★ ★
QUIET: ★ ★ ★ ★
CLEANLINESS: ★ ★ ★ ★
SECURITY: ★ ★ ★
SPACIOUSNESS: ★ ★ ★ ★

:: Key Information

ADDRESS: 745 Bliven Sherman Rd., Oxford, NY 13830

OPERATED BY: New York State Office of Parks, Recreation and Historic Preservation

CONTACT: 607-334-2718; nysparks .com/parks/76/details.aspx

OPEN: Early May–early October

SITES: 183

SITE AMENITIES: Picnic table and fire ring

ASSIGNMENT: Choose from available sites or reservations

REGISTRATION: On arrival or by reservation

FACILITIES: Water, flush toilets, showers, pay phone

PARKING: At site, maximum 2 vehicles, or designated lot for hike-in and boat-in sites

FEE: $15/night (plus $4/night for Fridays, Saturdays, and holidays)

ELEVATION: 1,685'

RESTRICTIONS:

■ **Pets:** Dogs on leash with proof of currently valid rabies vaccination

■ **Fires:** In fire rings only

■ **Alcohol:** At site

■ **Vehicles:** Up to 40'

■ **Other:** Quiet hours 10 p.m.–7 a.m.

■ **Reservations:** 2-night stay required

and are often set back deep into the trees. Sites located at forks in the road (such as 55) will see a bit too much traffic, but those along the outer edges (including 17 and 18) are wonderfully private. Sites 124–155, on the campground's northern edge, are more open and less appealing. Comfort stations, Dumpsters, and water spigots are scattered logically, so you need not worry about their proximity when choosing a site.

Campers will find plenty to keep themselves occupied in the park. A beach, basketball court, nature center, and a handful of swing sets will attract the kids. Motorboats are not permitted on 35-acre Bowman Lake, but kayaks, canoes, and rowboats are available to rent from the boathouse. If you plan to bring your own, make sure to obtain a permit from the park office. For a short walk, follow the small nature-trail loop around the lake and keep an eye out for white-tailed deer, red foxes, woodchucks, beavers, and a wide variety of birds. The park is a favorite of the Chenango Bird Club, which maintains an inventory of the avian population.

For more-extended hikes, set off on the two cross-country ski trails in the park (2 and 3 miles long), or the Kopac Trail, a 5-mile loop that passes by nearby Whaley Pond and Kopac Pond. The Finger Lakes Trail, a 560-mile thoroughfare that runs along the southern edge of the state from the Alleghenies to the Catskills, makes an appearance in the park, winding its way along the shore of the lake. Outside the park's boundaries, the state Department of Environmental Conservation maintains 11,000 acres of forested land, where even more adventures await outdoors enthusiasts.

Hunting is permitted in certain corners, so hikers should be sure to wear brightly colored clothing during autumn hunting seasons and should always stay on the trails. Central New York is legendary for its heavy snowfall, and in the wintertime, local cross-country skiers and snowmobilers descend on the park. It is a beautiful (if cold and blustery) time to visit, but unfortunately the park has discontinued its winter camping season. We hope that they consider reinstating it in the future.

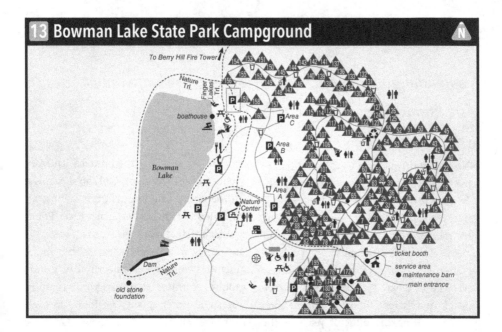

In the nearby village of Oxford, which was known for its bluestone mining in the 1800s, you can grab lunch, shop for antiques, and even catch a folk-music performance at the Night Eagle Cafe. However, you likely will not even need to leave the park, especially in the summer when the concession stand is selling camping supplies. Whether you will find it "paradise" or not, though, is up to you.

:: Getting There

From I-81 South, take Exit 6 and follow NY 12 North 25 miles to Oxford. Turn left on NY 220 West. Follow NY 220 for about 6 miles to Steere Road. Stay straight on Steere Road 1 mile and follow the signs to the park entrance, on the left.

GPS COORDINATES   N42° 30.983'   W75° 40.717'

14

Cherry Plain State Park

A splendid place to pitch a tent—serene, private, and little known in camping circles.

When traveling along CCC Dam Road to Cherry Plain State Park, many visitors probably don't think twice about what the CCC stands for, but without it the park wouldn't offer much for today's campers. President Franklin Roosevelt created the Civilian Conservation Corps in 1933 as part of the New Deal. The CCC gave young men a chance to work and helped improve the nation's resources during the difficult years of the Depression. For almost 10 years, different CCC groups worked around the country, often in flood control and in the establishment of state parks. In New York State, the Corps was instrumental in constructing the trails and buildings that are still used today throughout the park system. In Cherry Plain, they dammed Black Brook, creating Black River Pond. Though the park didn't open to the public until the early 1960s, the pond has always been its glimmering centerpiece.

Cherry Plain's modest 176 acres lie barely 20 miles east of Albany. Yet the park seems much farther from the capital, hidden away down country roads just north of the

Taconic Valley, along the border with Massachusetts and Vermont. Only 30 sites make up the entire campground, and almost all have views of the serene Black River Pond. For such a small park with a carry-in-carry-out policy, you may not expect too many amenities. But this is no primitive campground—comfort stations with running water and water spigots are found in each of the camping sections. A shower facility is also available and firewood is for sale at the registration booth.

The first group of sites is so pleasant that when we visited, our first impression was that they must be the tent sites. Surprisingly, they are reserved primarily for RVs and trailers, but we figure with gorgeous scenery in large supply, everyone deserves a fair share. Pine trees cast ample shade upon these nine sites, but they are a bit close together. A small stream runs along the edge of the section, with a charming wooden bridge crossing over it near site 1. Between sites 2 and 3 is the car-top boat launch, with a tiny dock. Sites 1–4 skirt the water's edge, and sites 5–9 are not far from the pond.

A recent expansion of the campground has brought a new collection of walk-in and overflow sites. Just across the bridge you will come upon a small parking lot flanked by trailer-friendly sites 10 and 11. From the parking lot, you can access walk-in sites 12–14. They offer a nice (and cheaper) respite from the motorized crowd, but for even

:: Ratings

BEAUTY: ★ ★ ★ ★ ★
PRIVACY: ★ ★ ★
QUIET: ★ ★ ★ ★ ★
CLEANLINESS: ★ ★ ★ ★
SECURITY: ★ ★ ★
SPACIOUSNESS: ★ ★ ★

:: Key Information

ADDRESS: 26 State Park Rd.,
P.O. Box 11, Cherry Plain, NY 12040

OPERATED BY: New York State Office
of Parks, Recreation and Historic
Preservation

CONTACT: 518-733-5400; nysparks
.com/parks/173/details.aspx

OPEN: Mid-May–early September

SITES: 30 tent sites, including
17 walk-in sites

SITE AMENITIES: Picnic table and
fire ring

ASSIGNMENT: Choose from available
sites or reservations

REGISTRATION: On arrival or by
reservation

FACILITIES: Water, flush toilets,
hot showers

PARKING: At site, maximum 2 vehicles

FEE: $15/night for drive-in, $12/night
for walk-in (plus $4/night for Fridays,
Saturdays, and holidays)

ELEVATION: 1,427'

RESTRICTIONS:

■ **Pets:** Dogs on leash with proof of
currently valid rabies vaccination

■ **Fires:** In fire rings only

■ **Alcohol:** At site

■ **Vehicles:** Up to 15'

■ **Other:** Quiet hours 10 p.m.–7 a.m.;
fires out by 11 p.m.

■ **Reservations:** 2-night stay required

more privacy and better access to the water, drive on to the next camping loop.

Skip sites 15 and 16, which sit along the edge of the day-use area parking lot, and keep going past sites 17–20, which are perched upon a small ledge. There are some views of the water here, but unless horseshoes is your game (there is a horseshoe pit nearby), drive to the parking lot next to site 21.

From the lot, a short path goes downhill to the water past a series of well-wooded sites, then back uphill to a comfort station and a few more sites; you can return to the lot along a service road. The closest site is 22, about a 15-yard walk on the well-maintained path. Sites 28–30 are nearest to the comfort station, convenient to be sure, but also a bit too far from the water's edge. Sites 24–27 are directly on the water, with 26 and 27 offering the most privacy. While there are not many sites to go around, this is nonetheless a splendid place to pitch a tent: serene, private, and little-known in camping circles.

It is among the nicest spots in all of New York State.

Back at the day-use area, you will find a sandy beach with a picnic pavilion. Swimmers enjoy the cool water of Black River Pond from late June to Labor Day, when lifeguards are on duty. Fishermen come for the bass, bullhead, and pickerel. Visitors can rent rowboats and paddleboats, but will have to leave any motorboats at home. Canoes and kayaks are a common sight, and the occasional small sailboat can be seen searching for a breeze. At the far western end of the water, bring a chair to sit near the dam's spillway, where you can crack open a book and spend a quiet summer day. Or, if you have a GPS unit (or even a smartphone), scour the grounds to find some of the geocaches hidden in the park.

Though the park is small compared with many others, there are plenty of recreational opportunities just beyond its borders. The Capital Region Wildlife Management Area

14 Cherry Plain State Park Campground

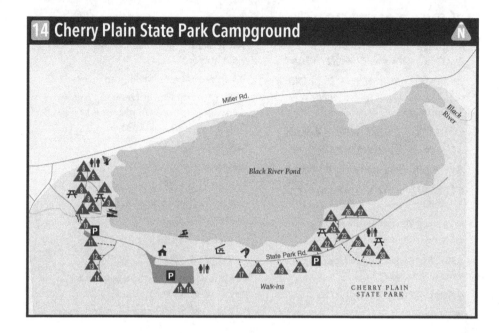

surrounds Cherry Plain with more than 4,000 acres of land and trails. If entering the park from the east, you may pass Black River Stables, which offer rides in the area, including some on bridle paths that pass through Cherry Plain.

The only trail contained entirely in the park is the half-mile hike to the Charcoal Kiln Site. Follow the signs from the main parking lot to see the remains of the stone oven where hardwoods were once covered with soil and set aflame. Deprived of oxygen, the resulting product, charcoal, was prized because it burns hotter and cleaner than wood. Today many campers still appreciate the ease of charcoal. Especially on a rainy evening or after a long day, it can make for a fast and easy dinner. But few would disagree that one of the best things about camping is sitting around a roaring campfire. Come to Cherry Plain in late May, when there's a nip in the air and spring flowers are bursting all around you, and you'll be happy you're here at the water's edge, beside a warm campfire, rather than home on the couch in front of the TV.

:: Getting There

From I-87 (New York State Thruway), take Exit 21A. Follow I-90 (Berkshire Spur) to Exit B3. Turn left on NY 22 North and follow it 20 miles. Turn left on CCC Dam Road. Follow CCC Dam Road 2.5 miles to the park entrance, on the left.

GPS COORDINATES   N42° 37.417'   W73° 24.567'

15

Delta Lake State Park

Go for a visit to Delta Lake State Park when the water level is low and, it is rumored, you may see rooftops of flooded homes.

In the history-rich Mohawk Valley, Delta Lake has quite a story of its own. It was once a natural lake, but when Ice Age glaciers covered the area and then retreated, it dried up. On the site of the ancient lake bed, the village of Delta was established and thrived, due in large part to its location on the Black River Canal, which was dug in the 1850s to connect the city of Rome to the Erie Canal. As the area grew, the need for a reservoir outweighed the need for a town. In 1912, the residents of Delta were relocated and the Mohawk River was dammed. A large body of water made a homecoming to the area after being gone for thousands of years, and now it had a name—Delta Lake. Fifty years passed before the state decided to create a park and take advantage of the recreational opportunities the reservoir offers. Go for a visit to Delta Lake State Park when the water level is low and, it is rumored, you may see rooftops of the flooded homes.

Lying on a peninsula that juts out from the southern shore, the park takes full advantage of its surrounding waters, including placing its campground directly on the lake. There is private development on other parts of the lake. Thankfully, it has not gotten out of hand, and although you can see some buildings along the shores, the views are still excellent. Entering the park, you pass the registration booth and then bear right to more than 100 camping sites.

Like most state-run campgrounds, Delta Lake State Park does not have electrical hookups, so some RV-ers may choose to motor on and plug in at the privately owned A-OK Campground & Marina, on the north shore of the lake. Still, trailers and pop-ups are inevitable, especially since the campground is a pleasant, well-run facility. When we visited, the park staff had placed flower boxes on the classic hewn park signs. With so many campgrounds in the state that look similar, sometimes it's the little things that make a difference.

Flat and made up of three main loops, the campground is located on a dead-end road. With a large proportion of waterfront sites available (nearly one out of every five), you have a good chance of landing a premium spot. No one waterfront site is better than any other, so choose any of the following: 8, 10, 12, 14, 16, 18, 20, 45, 46, 48, 50, 51, 53, 86, 88, 90, 92, 94, or 95. These book up fast on weekends (and cost a little extra), but the water is still easily accessible from interior sites.

In all three loops, tall hardwoods form a shady canopy and act as adequate

:: Ratings

BEAUTY: ★ ★ ★
PRIVACY: ★ ★
QUIET: ★ ★ ★
CLEANLINESS: ★ ★ ★
SECURITY: ★ ★ ★
SPACIOUSNESS: ★ ★ ★

:: Key Information

ADDRESS: 8797 NY 46, Rome, NY 13440

OPERATED BY: New York State Office of Parks, Recreation and Historic Preservation

CONTACT: 315-337-4670; nysparks .com/parks/66/details.aspx

OPEN: Early May–early October

SITES: 101

SITE AMENITIES: Picnic table and fire ring

ASSIGNMENT: Choose from available sites or reservations

REGISTRATION: On arrival or by reservation

FACILITIES: Water, flush toilets, hot showers, pay phone

PARKING: At site, maximum 2 vehicles

FEE: $15/night (plus $4/night for Fridays, Saturdays, and holidays and additional charge for waterfront sites)

ELEVATION: 555'

RESTRICTIONS:

▓ **Pets:** Dogs on leash with proof of currently valid rabies vaccination

▓ **Fires:** In fire rings only

▓ **Alcohol:** At site

▓ **Vehicles:** Up to 40'

▓ **Other:** Quiet hours 10 p.m.–7 a.m.

▓ **Reservations:** 2-night stay required

boundaries, but neighbors may be closer than some would wish. Loop A (sites 1–37) is the most exposed, with almost no understory to separate campers. Sites 38–70 make up Loop B. The center of this loop is a bit more cluttered, but more foliage sprouts from the forest floor, giving at least the feeling of privacy. Loop C (sites 71–101) is the smallest but also the most heavily wooded. It has only one comfort station (the other loops have two), but since it is quietly tucked away at the end of the camp road, this loop is our favorite. Dumpsters are placed conveniently throughout all loops, and the shower building, on the camp road between Loops B and C, is a short walk from just about any site.

The popular day-use area is filled with picnic areas, parking lots, a swimming beach, and a lake overlook. You can be sure it will be busy on hot summer days. Trails in the park connect the campground to three tiny ponds and over a land bridge to Treasure Island, a small chunk of land that has almost broken

off from the peninsula. A trailer boat launch is another big attraction, and anglers search the waters for bass, bullhead, northern pike, perch, trout, and walleye pike. The campground map helpfully includes locations where the various types of fish are commonly found and approximate depths of the water (65 feet at its deepest). All types of boats are allowed on the 2,560-acre lake, and if you have water access, you are welcome to launch canoes and kayaks directly from your site. Don't have a boat? Take a short drive to the previously mentioned A-OK Campground & Marina, where all varieties of watercraft are available for rent.

For a scenic view of the region, take a drive on the Black River Trail, a 111-mile byway that runs north along the western edge of the Adirondacks from Rome past Delta Lake to Ogdensburg on the St. Lawrence River. In the city of Rome, you can visit Fort Stanwix National Monument— built by the British during the French and Indian War and later occupied by Americans

15 Delta Lake State Park Campground

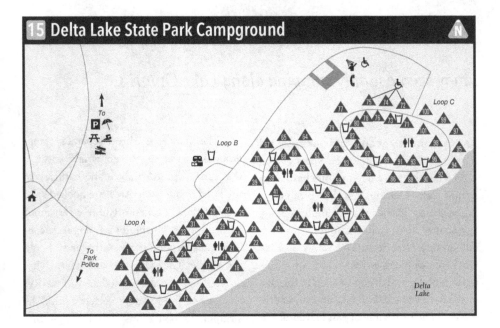

during the Revolutionary War. The fort protected the Oneida Carrying Place, a 3-mile portage between the Mohawk River and Wood Creek. It was an essential trail for transporting goods and news (not to mention viruses), as early travelers journeyed the Northeast's inland waterways. Today Fort Stanwix sits at a busy intersection, its simple log construction contrasting sharply with the surrounding big-box stores and chain restaurants. It's a fascinating place to visit for an afternoon.

:: Getting There

Take I-90 (New York State Thruway) to Exit 32, Westmoreland/Rome. Follow NY 233 North 7 miles to Rome, then follow NY 46 North 6 miles to the park entrance.

GPS COORDINATES   N43° 17.417'   W75° 24.900'

16

Fair Haven Beach State Park

Enjoy scenic family camping along Lake Ontario.

As the most-recent glacier receded from New York about 10,000 years ago, it carved out the 7,340-square-mile basin that is now Lake Ontario. Another product of the receding glacier was drumlins—long, egg-shaped hills that are found throughout upstate New York. The waves of Lake Ontario have been eroding these drumlins to form bluffs, which can be seen to the east of the park's beach. The lake and these dramatic bluffs form some of Fair Haven Beach State Park's unique features.

Lake Ontario forms Fair Haven Beach State Park's northern edge, and Little Sodus Bay the park's eastern boundary. Overnight docks and a public boat launch are available in Little Sodus Bay and provide boating access to Lake Ontario. The remainder of the park is bordered along its southern and western edges by Sterling Pond and Sterling Marsh. Given the quantity and diversity of the park's waterscape, fishing, boating, and birding make up the majority of activities available at the park. Swimming is allowed only in designated areas when a lifeguard is on duty.

:: Ratings

BEAUTY: ★ ★ ★
PRIVACY: ★ ★ ★
QUIET: ★ ★ ★
CLEANLINESS: ★ ★ ★
SECURITY: ★ ★ ★
SPACIOUSNESS: ★ ★ ★

The park has three separate campgrounds as well as 36 cabins and cottages that can be rented. Cabins and cottages, in the Pond Shore Cabin Area, are booked solid most of the season and require reservations far in advance. The Bluff Camping Area contains 44 large pull-up sites with electric hookups for RVs. The Lakeview Camping Area has 14 sites and can accommodate various RVs and trailers, but has only 2 electric sites. The Drumlin Camping Area has 126 sites that range from tent-only sites to 30-foot RV/trailer sites; none have electric hookups.

The Bluff camping sites are essentially for RVs—they are surrounded by trees and have no views of the lake, pond, or marsh. The Lakeview sites sit atop the bluff and offer expansive views of Lake Ontario. The sites are closely spaced and consequently provide little privacy. Both the Bluff and Lakeview sites have access to comfort stations and potable water, but there are no showers in the Lakeview area. Campers interested in views of the lake should consider the Lakeview area, but the majority of sites for tent campers are in the Drumlin camping area.

A canopy of conifers and mixed hardwoods shades the Drumlin Camping Area, which is served by three comfort stations including showers. Potable-water stations are available throughout the area, as are a centrally located Dumpster and a recycling station. Sites along the outside western edge of the campground are shielded from the park's main road by a thin row of trees, and

:: Key Information

ADDRESS: NY 104A, P.O. Box 16, Fair Haven, NY 13064

OPERATED BY: New York State Office of Parks, Recreation and Historic Preservation

CONTACT: 315-947-5205; nysparks .com/parks/12/details.aspx

OPEN: April-mid-October

SITES: 185 tent sites, including 46 electric sites

SITE AMENITIES: Picnic table, fire ring

ASSIGNMENT: Choose from available sites or reservations

REGISTRATION: 3 p.m.-9 p.m.

FACILITIES: Picnic areas, pavilion, potable water, flush toilets, park store, boat rentals, boat launch, showers

PARKING: At site

FEE: $15/night Drumlin Camping Area, $20-$25/night Lakeview and Bluff Camping Areas (extra $4/night on Fridays, Saturdays, and holidays). See website for cabin and cottage fees (click "Fees and Rates" on the home page).

ELEVATION: 384'

RESTRICTIONS:

■ **Pets:** Dogs on leash with proof of currently valid rabies vaccination

■ **Fires:** In fire rings only

■ **Alcohol:** Allowed

■ **Vehicles:** RVs and trailers limited to specific sites

■ **Other:** Quiet hours 10 p.m.-7 a.m.

■ **Reservations:** 2-night stay required

views of the park's waterscape are absent. Interior sites near the western edge are denser than those along the edge and also lack views of the waterscape. Though the surrounding understory is thick, brief glimpses of the pond and marsh are available to interior sites along the eastern edge. These sites are also fairly dense and well within view of nearby sites. The exterior loop of the campground road provides access to the more desirable sites, most of which are tent-only (with a few for small trailers). The loop road descends toward the marsh. This change in elevation, combined with the addition of a dense understory, isolates these sites along the eastern edge from the rest of the campground. Increased spaciousness, thicker woods, and greater distances between sites complement this privacy. Views of Sterling Marsh are greatly improved here, with some sites lying on the water's edge. The last few sites along this loop share views of Sterling Pond as well as the marsh.

The park has numerous picnic tables, comfort stations, and grills for public use. Near the East Beach, look for a recreation hall, snack bar, bathhouse, camp store, and boat and bicycle rentals. Also within this park are several playgrounds and a ball field, making this park very family friendly. Two short hiking trails provide an alternative for those wishing to forgo the park's main activities. Wildlife in the area is most notably beaver, muskrat, a variety of waterfowl, and migratory birds; fortunate visitors might even catch a glimpse of an otter.

Wildlife enthusiasts and hikers looking for more-remote trails should visit Sterling Lakeshore Park and Nature Center, a short drive north from the park. This park also features glacial bluffs, guided nature walks, and diverse waterscapes.

Long-distance hikers and cyclists may want to try either the Cato–Fair Haven Trail or the Cayuga Hojak Trail, both of which are converted railroad beds and offer long and

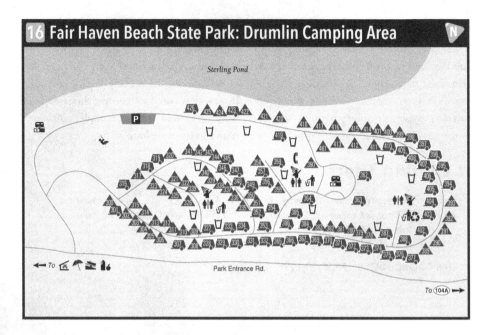

16 Fair Haven Beach State Park: Drumlin Camping Area

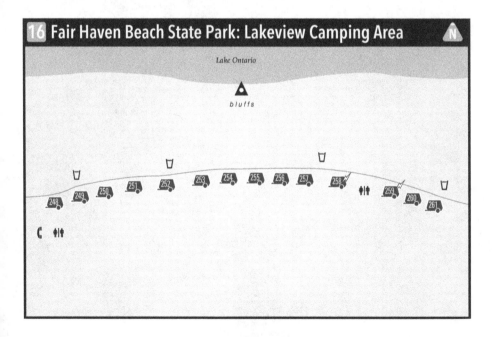

16 Fair Haven Beach State Park: Lakeview Camping Area

mostly flat routes. Access to both is within Fair Haven. Visitors during the summer may also want to consider the Sterling Renaissance Festival, open weekends from July to mid-August. Travelers wishing to view more of Lake Ontario—with its historic battlegrounds, forts, lighthouses, vineyards, and other attractions—can drive, bike, or walk along the Seaway Trail, a 454-mile byway that traverses the northern edge of New York State and offers a pleasant alternative to the interstate.

:: Getting There

From I-90 (New York State Thruway), take Exit 34A, I-481 North, toward Oswego. Follow I-481 for 6.7 miles until it changes to NY 481 North. Continue 20 miles and turn left on NY 176/NY 3. Follow NY 3 for 11.7 miles and turn left on NY 104A. Follow NY 104A for 4 miles. The park entrance is on the right.

GPS COORDINATES   N43° 19.117'   W76° 41.767'

17

Glimmerglass State Park

In Cooper's classic stories, set during the French and Indian War, the sparkling Otsego Lake is known as Glimmerglass.

The family-friendly campground at Glimmerglass State Park lies in the heart of New York's Leatherstocking region, a hilly collection of farms and small towns named after James Fenimore Cooper's five novels that together are known as *The Leatherstocking Tales*. They include *The Pioneers, The Deerslayer,* and, most famously, *The Last of the Mohicans*. In Cooper's classic stories, set during the French and Indian War, the sparkling Otsego Lake is known as Glimmerglass. Though born in New Jersey, Cooper spent his childhood and formative years in this area when his family moved to what would become Cooperstown, and the area greatly influenced his writing.

Similar in shape and geology to the Finger Lakes, Otsego is long and narrow, cutting a sliver in the land for 8 miles. On the northern end of the lake is Glimmerglass State Park; at the southern end is Cooperstown, founded by and named after James Fenimore Cooper's father. Cooperstown, as most people know, is home to the Baseball Hall of Fame. Local lore tells how baseball was invented in the town, but the origin of the sport has been debated for years. Whatever the true story is, the region offers an appealing combination of history and recreation, and Glimmerglass is a fine place for tent campers to begin their explorations.

The manicured lawns and rolling hills of the park are home to two separate camping areas. Two loops make up the main camping area, with 37 standard, if a bit small, sites. Towering fir trees divide and shade the spaces, but no understory provides privacy. A field separates the two loops, and on busy weekends children collect there to play ball and reach for the skies on the swing set. Crowds abate during the week, and walk-ins can easily find openings. We prefer sites 20, 21, or the private 36 over the bare and exposed 33–35, which are more suited to trailers. The comfort stations with showers are clean, well maintained, and located near the garbage and recycling centers. Follow campground procedures for refuse—raccoons are common in the park and not too picky about what they have for dinner.

Near Beaver Pond, on the northern end of the park, is the separate primitive-camping area with six available sites. Although you'll find only one water spigot, and Porta-Potties provide the only "comfort station," this is where you will often see tents in the park. Two of the most popular sites are 45 and 46, located near the edge of a small pond. Not far from site 45 you'll see a lean-to, which

:: Ratings

BEAUTY: ★ ★ ★
PRIVACY: ★ ★
QUIET: ★ ★ ★
CLEANLINESS: ★ ★ ★ ★
SECURITY: ★ ★ ★
SPACIOUSNESS: ★ ★

:: Key Information

ADDRESS: 1527 CR 31, Cooperstown, NY 13326

OPERATED BY: New York State Office of Parks, Recreation and Historic Preservation

CONTACT: 607-547-8662; nysparks .com/parks/28/details.aspx

OPEN: Mid-May–early October (some walk-in sites available year-round)

SITES: 43 (6 primitive sites at Beaver Pond Area)

SITE AMENITIES: Picnic table, grill, and fire ring

ASSIGNMENT: Choose from available sites or reservations

REGISTRATION: On arrival or by reservation

FACILITIES: Water, showers, flush toilets (only pit toilet at walk-in sites)

PARKING: At site, maximum 2 vehicles, or central lot for walk-in sites

FEE: $15/night for most sites and $12/ night for primitive sites (plus $4/night for Fridays, Saturdays, and holidays)

ELEVATION: 1,276'

RESTRICTIONS:

■ **Pets:** Dogs on leash with proof of currently valid rabies vaccination

■ **Fires:** In fire rings only

■ **Alcohol:** At site

■ **Vehicles:** Up to 30'

■ **Other:** Quiet hours 10 p.m.–8 a.m.

■ **Reservations:** 2-night stay required

doubles as a warming hut during the ice-skating season. Sites 44 and 47–49 feature low foliage, bushes, and small, young trees. Sites 46 and 48 offer the best shade.

Winter camping is allowed at Beaver Pond but is rare, according to camp staff (only three or four campers each season). Perhaps this would be a great place to try out cold-weather gear, but be sure to call ahead. If you decide to visit in the winter, the park's many activities include ice-skating, ice fishing, snowshoeing, cross-country skiing, and snow tubing.

In the warmer months, the beach attracts visitors with its lifeguards, pavilion, picnic shelters, snack bar, first-aid station, ball fields, and playgrounds. Water enthusiasts will find a car-top boat launch at the park, and canoes and kayaks are a common sight, but those with larger vessels will have to drive to Cooperstown for the trailer boat launch. Anglers can use the shoreline or boats to fish for lake and brown trout, smallmouth and

largemouth bass, coho salmon, brown bullhead, yellow perch, or chain pickerel. Several trails loop through the park, including a short nature trail near Beaver Pond and the longer Woodland Trail, both of which attract birders and locals looking for an afternoon jaunt. The orange-blazed, 2.5-mile Sleeping Lion Trail, named for the creature Mount Wellington is said to resemble, starts behind Hyde Hall and skirts the edge of the peak.

Within the park is a national and state historic site, consisting of Hyde Hall and its many outbuildings. The 50-room Classical Revival mansion is the centerpiece of a property once owned by George Clark. The state bought the land from his descendants in the 1960s. Today, visitors can tour Hyde Hall daily in the summer, but only after paying an entrance fee.

If you are not game for a trip to the Baseball Hall of Fame, perhaps you would like to take in a little opera before a night of camping. Just down the road on Route 80, the

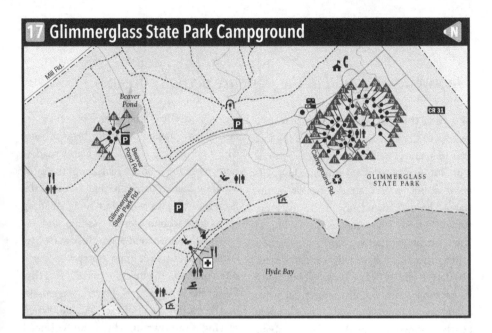

17 Glimmerglass State Park Campground

renowned Glimmerglass Opera holds shows at the Alice Busch Opera Theater four or five days a week during the summer. Make a full day of it and check out other local attractions, such as the Fenimore Art Museum, Farmers' Museum, and Ommegang Brewery.

Glimmerglass has much to offer campers. Even if you're not a rugged adventurer in the mold of Cooper's famed character Hawkeye, this bit of central New York offers a fine getaway for a family looking for a bit of fresh air.

:: Getting There

From I-90 (New York State Thruway), take Exit 25A to I-88. Follow I-88 to Exit 24, Duanesburg/Cooperstown. Follow NY 20 West for about 36 miles. In the town of East Springfield, take a left on CR 31 South. Follow CR 31 South 4 miles to the park entrance, on the right.

GPS COORDINATES   N42° 47.133'   W74° 51.683'

18

Green Lakes State Park

The two lakes found in the park are actually green.

The first thing that surprises first-time visitors to Green Lakes State Park is the fact that its name is neither an exaggeration nor a quaint evocation of the surrounding wilderness, but an accurate description of the water: the two lakes found in the park are actually green. The smaller one is Round Lake, an almost perfect circle of emerald water surrounded by heavily wooded slopes. The larger one is Green Lake—about twice its neighbor's size and also round, but with a long spur that juts out and ends at a sandy beach. Formed by Ice Age glaciers about 14,000 years ago, both are meromictic, a rare type of lake (there are only a few others in the United States) where the surface and bottom waters do not mix. They are small, but astoundingly deep—it's nearly 200 feet to the bottom of each! These factors, along with the presence of calcium carbonate, cause mainly green light to be reflected by the water, producing the odd but beautiful color that intrigues and delights those who take to the trails along the lakes' shores.

The lakes are indeed gorgeous. We wish we could say the same about the park's campground. Divided into two looping sections, the sites at Green Lakes are grassy,

clean, and adequately large, but they are also poorly shaded and offer little privacy. The first section along the camp road is known as Pine Wood, which is not the most accurate name. There are pine trees on the far edges of sites 1–64, but none dividing them. The second section, Rolling Hills, is more aptly named and contains sites 65–132. Exterior sites are set upon grassy slopes and often overlook the mix of tents and RVs that fill up the campground. Electric sites make up the northern end of each section. When placing a reservation, which you will need on summer weekends, skip those and opt for any site where fewer neighboring sites are reserved. This seems obvious, but we say it because no particular site stands out, and you are most likely to enjoy your stay if you have more privacy.

The campground features the typical amenities, including large comfort stations, conveniently distributed water spigots, and even small jungle gyms in the center of each section. A nature center in the Pine Wood section is open throughout the summer and offers programs for youngsters. And just south of Pine Woods, a series of seven rustic cabins are available to rent. They are nothing fancy, but a few are set along the edge of a cliff and look down onto the waters of Round Lake.

We don't mean to paint the campground as inadequate, but compared with the rest of the park, it is the place where you will want to spend the least amount of your time. Green Lakes is quite simply one of the nicest parks in the New York

:: Ratings

BEAUTY: ★ ★
PRIVACY: ★ ★
QUIET: ★ ★ ★
CLEANLINESS: ★ ★ ★
SECURITY: ★ ★ ★ ★
SPACIOUSNESS: ★ ★

:: Key Information

ADDRESS: 7900 Green Lakes Rd., Fayetteville, NY 13066

OPERATED BY: New York State Office of Parks, Recreation and Historic Preservation

CONTACT: 315-637-6111; nysparks .com/parks/172/details.aspx

OPEN: Mid-May–early October

SITES: 132

SITE AMENITIES: Picnic table and fire ring

ASSIGNMENT: Choose from available sites or reservations

REGISTRATION: On arrival or by reservation

FACILITIES: Water, flush toilets, hot showers, pay phone

PARKING: At site, maximum 2 vehicles

FEE: $15/night (plus $4/night for Fridays, Saturdays, and holidays)

ELEVATION: 469'

RESTRICTIONS:

■ **Pets:** Dogs on leash with proof of currently valid rabies vaccination

■ **Fires:** In fire rings only

■ **Alcohol:** At site

■ **Vehicles:** Up to 40'

■ **Other:** Quiet hours 10 p.m.–7 a.m.; no private boats on lakes; swimming allowed from Memorial Day to Labor Day

■ **Reservations:** 2-night stay required

system—arguably, it has the state's best facilities and presents the best range of activities in the Syracuse area.

The lakes are, of course, the stars of the park. The beach entices locals on summer days and is worth visiting, but you will first want to stroll along the trails that follow the lakes' outer rims. The water is very dangerous away from the beach. Take the NO SWIMMING signs seriously, and keep your feet on the impeccably maintained path. This is where the local high school's national-championship-winning cross-country team trains in the summer and where many a dog walker comes to escape the bland, paved roads of the suburbs—and for good reason. As the trail approaches the water's edge, notice how the shore drops off suddenly, almost as if it were a bottomless pit. American Indians and early European settlers believed just that. Scientists still study the lower depths, where evidence of ancient plants and animals may exist.

There is more to the park, though, than just the lakes. Make sure to stop by the campground office and pick up a map to the park's 10 miles of trails. A trail leaving from Pine Woods and through Rolling Hills will take you south down a hill and into the surrounding woods, some of the only old-growth forest in the region. Follow another trail west from Rolling Hills and you will find yourself among the fields of Farmer's Hill. This is the site of a former farm and was purchased by the park in the 1980s. Mountain bikers looking for gentle, scenic pedaling would be hard-pressed to find better trails elsewhere. If you do bring your bike, pay attention to signs: a handful of the park's trails are designated for foot traffic only. This includes the wonderfully named Hernia Hill Bypass, which only masochists would want to tackle on a bike anyway.

Golf, whether traditional or played with Frisbees, is available to those who seek it. The 18 holes on the southeast end of the

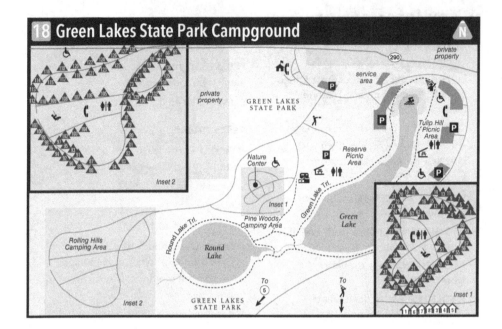

18 Green Lakes State Park Campground

park constitute one of the area's best public courses. And the clubhouse, with its outdoor restaurant, serves up lovely views of Green Lake to go with burgers and sandwiches. The disc-golf course, near Pine Woods, is a confidence-booster for those of us with laughable golf swings but a great Frisbee toss.

In the interest of disclosure, two of this book's authors grew up in a house literally yards from the border of Green Lakes State Park and spent their childhoods exploring its 1,756 acres. It is hard to avoid some nostalgia, but we must say that after traveling throughout the state and seeing many wonderful campgrounds and parks, we still keep coming back to visit. We hope that after spending a weekend at Green Lakes, you'll do the same.

:: Getting There

From I-90 (New York State Thruway), take Exit 34 to I-481 South. Follow I-481 South 1 mile to the Kirkville Road exit. Follow Kirkville Road 1 mile to Fremont Road and turn right. After 1 mile, turn left on CR 290; follow 3 miles to the park entrance, on the right.

GPS COORDINATES N43° 03.583' W75° 58.283'

19

Max V. Shaul State Park

*A great example of the advantages of a small park
with only a handful of campsites.*

Even though it's a bit of a drive from the highway, and even though the signs along the way make you think you're going in circles (are you in Fulton, West Fulton, or Fultonham?), it is certainly a pleasant journey through the Schoharie Valley to Max V. Shaul State Park. If you do make it to the park, you'll be rewarded with a peaceful, isolated camping experience. This small park sits among the rolling hills of the historic Leatherstocking region, just north of the Catskills and about an hour's drive west of Albany. Although recreational opportunities are limited within its 54 acres, it is a great place to camp and enjoy a little quiet.

After you go through the gate and past the unassuming park office, stay right on the main camp road, and make your way through the hardwoods—lush and green in summer and bursting with reds and yellows in fall. Appropriately, maple-leaf markers designate the 30 nicely shaded sites distributed along two joined loops. A rough paved road winds uphill through the first loop, with sites numbered 1–22. Sites on the loop's exterior are the most desirable. They are flat and on the small side, but spacious enough for a tent or two. Set back at least 15 yards from the road and enveloped by thick circles of trees, sites 3, 4, 13, and 21 stand out as the best. Sites 17–20 sit close to the road, but are the most widely spaced from each other. Located along the park's outer boundary, they are also bordered by a steep rise to Toe Path Mountain. Site 17 is wheelchair-accessible. Water spigots are well placed throughout the loop, and the centrally located comfort station is relatively easy to find in the dark.

Rarely does the park reach capacity, and unless you want a specific site, reservations are recommended only on holiday weekends. None of the sites could be considered bad, but the second loop (sites 23–30) is certainly the least-private corner of the campground. These spaces are right next to new comfort stations, a swing set, a picnic area, and a series of small parking areas. This may be appealing to families with little ones or to people expecting visitors. A group-camping area opens up behind site 30, where NY 30 meets Panther Creek. If you camp here, you may have a family reunion or perhaps some Scouts as neighbors.

This park differs from many state-run campgrounds in that it has no major day-use facilities. Picnicking may attract the occasional family, but campers primarily use the park. A basketball hoop, small playground, softball diamond, and horseshoe pit keep

:: Ratings

BEAUTY: ★ ★ ★
PRIVACY: ★ ★ ★ ★
QUIET: ★ ★ ★ ★ ★
CLEANLINESS: ★ ★ ★ ★
SECURITY: ★ ★ ★ ★
SPACIOUSNESS: ★ ★ ★ ★

:: Key Information

ADDRESS: NY 30, P.O. Box 23, Fultonham, NY 12071

OPERATED BY: New York State Office of Parks, Recreation and Historic Preservation

CONTACT: 518-827-4711; nysparks .com/parks/94/details.aspx

OPEN: Late May–early September

SITES: 30

SITE AMENITIES: Picnic table and fire ring

ASSIGNMENT: Choose from available sites or reservations

REGISTRATION: On arrival or by reservation

FACILITIES: Water, flush toilets, hot showers

PARKING: At site, maximum 2 vehicles

FEE: $15/night (plus $4/night for Fridays, Saturdays, and holidays)

ELEVATION: 708'

RESTRICTIONS:

■ **Pets:** Dogs on leash with proof of currently valid rabies vaccination

■ **Fires:** In fire rings only

■ **Alcohol:** At site

■ **Vehicles:** Up to 30'

■ **Other:** Quiet hours 10 p.m.–7 a.m.; carry out all trash

■ **Reservations:** 2-night stay required

people entertained. A recently added trail helps kayakers and canoeists reach nearby Schoharie Creek. In general, this is not a destination that draws campers from many miles away.

You may fish in Panther Creek across NY 30; just stay along the sections inside the park boundary, as much of the creek runs through private property. Outside of Max V. Shaul State Park, anglers will find several other options. Brown trout stocks Schoharie Creek, which runs through the center of the valley. Largemouth bass fills Looking Glass Pond, an artificial body of water in Fulton.

A trail starting near site 16 leads out of the campground for a short hike up Toe Path Mountain. Campers arriving from the north may spot another popular hiking destination known as Vroman's Nose, where the land rises dramatically 600 feet from the valley floor. The short, steep trail is part of the Long Path, a 335-mile trail running from the New Jersey end of the George Washington Bridge north along the Palisades and through the

Shawangunk and Catskill Mountains, finally ending at John Boyd Thacher Park outside of Albany. This slice of the path offers great, unobstructed views of the valley.

Nearby attractions include other state parks, historical sites, and caves. Tours of the perennially popular Howe Caverns leave daily and showcase an underground river. Not far from Howe, the lesser-known Secret Caverns is smaller but contains many oddly shaped formations and a 100-foot underground waterfall that should delight all ages. The cool year-round underground temperature of 52°F makes both caves great places to visit on a hot summer day. Or cool off at Mine Kill State Park, which campers can enter free during the length of their stay at Max V. Shaul (be sure to bring your camping receipt). You can hike its trails, visit its waterfall, and take advantage of its bathing complex, complete with wading, diving, and Olympic-size swimming pools. Finally, Cooperstown and the Baseball Hall of Fame (about an hour's drive away) are the

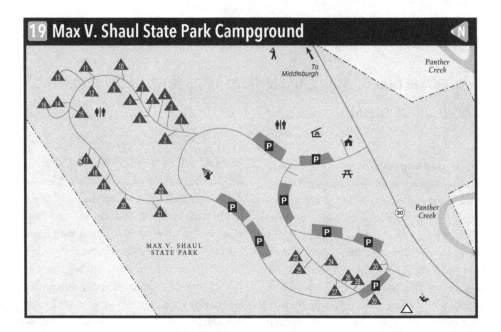

19 Max V. Shaul State Park Campground

centerpieces of the surrounding Leather-stocking region's long and rich history.

As for Max V. Shaul State Park, its story is a little more recent. The land was donated by and named after a local farmer and involved citizen. The park opened in 1960 and was rededicated upon Max Shaul's death in 1980. It remains a great example of the advantages of a small park with only a handful of campsites. Although a number of things keep campers busy in the area, the real attraction of the campground is the quiet. Even though you may not be pitching your tent in wilderness that stretches for miles, you will still feel that you have the woods to yourself.

:: Getting There

From I-88, take Exit 22 (Cobleskill/Middleburgh) to NY 145 South. Follow NY 145 about 8 miles to the town of Middleburgh. Turn right on NY 30 and follow it south about 6 miles. The park entrance is on the right.

GPS COORDINATES   N42° 32.783'   W74° 24.617'

20

Moreau Lake State Park

Moreau is one of many kettle-hole lakes formed by glaciers carving out the land.

Most day-trippers come to Moreau Lake for the main attraction—a large, sandy beach in a region where such things are in short supply. A few picnickers and sunbathers even venture out and around the park's Mud Pond to enjoy a nature trail. But stay a night or more and you'll get a chance to know a third body of water in the park—the Hudson River. Carving a winding path through the park's northeast corner, the river passes through breathtaking scenery and by several primitive boat-in campsites. Moreau Lake State Park is technically part of the Adirondack foothills, the "blue line" on maps that marks the border of the Adirondack Park. The latter is less than 2 miles to the north, but Moreau is a distinct park on its own, and its clear waters, green woods, and pleasant camping loops will surely satisfy campers looking for an easily accessible bit of nature.

Moreau Lake is a nearly 4-hour drive from Manhattan, but perhaps more important, just 10 minutes from the New York Thruway. Visitors intent on getting to the beach may never even see the campground.

:: Ratings

BEAUTY: ★ ★ ★
PRIVACY: ★ ★ ★
QUIET: ★ ★ ★
CLEANLINESS: ★ ★ ★
SECURITY: ★ ★ ★ ★
SPACIOUSNESS: ★ ★ ★

Beyond the park office and registration booth, the camp road splits, leading left to the beach and day-use facilities and right to the campground. Pick up ice and firewood at the office. When we camped here, the firewood was distributed in burlap wood bags (with a small deposit per bag), which are an environmentally friendly alternative to the standard shrink-wrap plastic that so often litters sites. After registering, follow the main road past the wooden guard posts that mark the steep drop to lake's edge. Some of the seven camping loops flank each other and some skirt the edge of a metal fence that marks the border of the park with Mountain Road. Campers share just one shower building, located between Loops E and F, but comfort stations are well distributed in the center of each loop.

Mixed hardwoods and firs shade the sites, which will fill up with an equal mix of RVs, pop-up trailers, and tents. Reservations are a necessity during summer weekends. Loop A features flat, roomy, nicely wooded spaces, and was the least crowded when we visited. Loop B is smaller, with some of the best-spaced sites, but houses can be seen through the trees, especially when the trees lose their leaves, spoiling the illusion of being deep in the woods. You'll find Loops C and D on rough roads up a steep hill from the lake, with spotty views of the water through the trees. Some campers mistakenly think they are getting prime lakefront spots when

:: Key Information

ADDRESS: 605 Old Saratoga Rd., Gansevoort, NY 12831

OPERATED BY: New York State Office of Parks, Recreation and Historic Preservation

CONTACT: 518-793-0511; nysparks .com/parks/150/details.aspx

OPEN: Early May–early October

SITES: 148 (including 7 wheelchair-accessible sites) plus 2 boat-in sites

SITE AMENITIES: Picnic table and fire ring

ASSIGNMENT: Choose from available sites or reservations

REGISTRATION: On arrival or by reservation

FACILITIES: Water, flush toilets, showers, pay phone

PARKING: At site, maximum 2 vehicles

FEE: $15/night (plus $4/night on Fridays, Saturdays, and holidays)

ELEVATION: 215'

RESTRICTIONS:

■ **Pets:** Dogs on leash with proof of currently valid rabies vaccination

■ **Fires:** In fire rings only

■ **Alcohol:** At site

■ **Vehicles:** Up to 40'

■ **Other:** Quiet hours 10 p.m.–7 a.m.; no motorboats

■ **Reservations:** 2-night stay required

they reserve these sites, but they are a nice option nonetheless. Site 72 in Loop D has grown to be one of the largest, evidence that equipment placed on the edge of the site reduces the surrounding vegetation over time. Loops F and G are well removed from the rest, but the sites are more congested—and again, views of a nearby residential development can be an annoyance.

To really get away from it all, bring a sturdy boat and access one of the two primitive boat-in sites on the Hudson. Bennie Brook and the deceptively named Sherman Island (actually near, not on, an island) are such nice places to camp that the park plans to develop several more riverside sites in the future. The sites are little more than a fire ring in a clearing—sorry, no picnic tables or toilets here. Reservations are not available and they fill up on a first-come, first-serve basis. But it is not a matter of making a mad dash down the river. Campers must first obtain a free overnight-parking pass from the campground office and use one of the

two boat ramps on Spier Falls Road to access the river from inside the park.

The park has built a causeway footbridge to separate the two sections of the semicolon-shaped lake. Moreau is one of many kettle-hole lakes formed by glaciers carving out the land. Past the first of the park's two full-service rental cottages is the beach complex, with parking, designated swimming area, store, snack bar, and nature center, which hosts daily events in summer. Whether you want to rent fishing poles and tackle or umbrellas and lounge chairs, you can find them here. No motorboats are allowed on the lake, but this is not necessarily the quietest corner of the park—the beach gets very busy on warm days.

More than 20 miles of trails crisscross the Palmertown Mountain Range, a series of 1,000-foot bumps that border the southern side of the Hudson. All 12 trails are clearly marked, but we recommend picking up a topographic map at the park office—well worth the small fee. These are

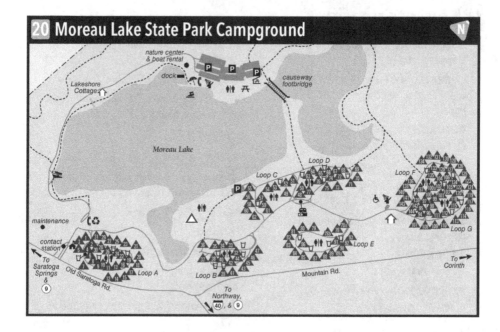

20 Moreau Lake State Park Campground

multiuse trails, so watch out for mountain bikes. Trails range in distance, starting with the short but steep Overlook Trail and its great views of the lake. The Nature Trail is just over 1 mile, with an interpretive loop that runs over the causeway, through Loop D, and reaches Mud Pond. Another option is the Western Ridge Trail, which climbs 5 miles to Spring Overlook. Enjoy the view of the Northern Luzerne Mountain Range

across the bend in the river and keep an eye out for hawks and eagles.

Moreau Lake is a great place to stay while exploring the surrounding area. Twenty miles to the north is Lake George, with its many recreational activities; 10 miles to the south is the famed horse track at Saratoga Springs. Thankfully, campers can avoid the Lake George crowds and will be betting on a sure thing by pitching a tent at Moreau Lake.

:: Getting There

From I-87 (Adirondack Northway), take Exit 17S, South Glen Falls, to NY 9 South. Take the first right on Old Saratoga Road. Drive less than 1 mile to the park entrance, on the right.

GPS COORDINATES N43°13.800' W73° 42.400'

21

Whetstone Gulf State Park

Explore the Lesser Wilderness while camping at the outlet of a 3-mile gorge.

Whetstone Gulf is located between two of New York's greatest natural resources, the Tug Hill plateau and the Adirondacks. Whereas the Iroquois referred to the Adirondack region as the "Greater Wilderness," they called the Tug Hill region the "Lesser Wilderness." Settlers would eventually replace this misleading title, choosing "Tug Hill" instead. The Tug Hill area is made up of 150,000 acres of unbroken hardwood forest with many creeks, brooks, and streams. Gorges—sometimes locally called *gulfs*—are cut by these running waters, and Whetstone Gulf is a truly amazing example.

Whetstone Gulf has served as a recreation area since the 1800s, and was formally acquired as a state park in the 1920s. Improvements by the New York State Conservation Department and the federal Civilian Conservation Corps followed during the 1930s and again after World War II. Evidence of their hard work can be seen today, including a man-made beach, bridges, trails, and plantings of red pine, a fast-growing species seen throughout the park.

:: Ratings

BEAUTY: ★ ★
PRIVACY: ★ ★ ★
QUIET: ★ ★ ★
CLEANLINESS: ★ ★ ★
SECURITY: ★ ★
SPACIOUSNESS: ★ ★ ★

These tall pines provide shade and a bit of privacy for 51 of the 62 campsites. The spacious sites (along with water spigots and multiple Dumpsters for recycling) are located along several one-way loops. Three comfort stations and one shower serve the area. Dense pines and understory brush screen sites along the north edge of the campground from the main park road. Most interior sites are openly visible to each other, and though they provide less privacy than those along the edge, the dense trees give the area a woodland atmosphere rather than an open campground. Sites along the east and south edges are more secluded, private, and spacious. The southern sites are farther apart and benefit from a dense understory that has begun to grow as the native hardwood forest encroaches. Each site has a stone fire pit with grill top, gravel drive, and adequate space for spreading out. You'll find the 20 sites with electric hookups primarily along the easternmost loop (sites 3–17) and along the interior loop.

Situated off the parking area near the beach and Whetstone Creek, the last six sites are essentially overflow sites. These sites are wide open, directly next to each other, and adjacent to much of the park's foot traffic and other activities. Reservations are recommended for weekends and holidays, as most sites are booked well in advance. Weekday campers can expect available sites without reservations.

:: Key Information

ADDRESS: 6065 West Rd., Lowville, NY 13367

OPERATED BY: New York State Office of Parks, Recreation and Historic Preservation

CONTACT: 315-376-6630; nysparks .com/parks/92/details.aspx

OPEN: Memorial Day–mid-September

SITES: 62 tent sites, including 20 electric sites

SITE AMENITIES: Stone fire pit, picnic table

ASSIGNMENT: Choose from available sites or reservations

REGISTRATION: 3 p.m.–9 p.m.

FACILITIES: Picnic tables, beach, bathhouse, pavilion, potable water, flush toilets, showers

PARKING: At site

FEE: $15/night (extra $4/night on Fridays, Saturdays, and holidays)

ELEVATION: 1,300'

RESTRICTIONS:

■ **Pets:** Dogs on leash with proof of currently valid rabies vaccination

■ **Fires:** In fire pits only

■ **Alcohol:** Allowed

■ **Vehicles:** RVs and trailers allowed

■ **Other:** Quiet hours 10 p.m.–7 a.m.

■ **Reservations:** 2-night stay required; 1-night reservations available if reserved within 3 days of visit

The park's swimming area, created by the damming of Whetstone Creek, is just a short walk from the main campsite area. You can reach a playground, a bathhouse, and a recreation building directly from the beach. Past the beach and across a short bridge is the park's picnic area, accessed along a road that follows Whetstone Creek up the gorge. You'll find plenty of picnic tables and charcoal grills along this meandering road, but the wooded views of the gulf at this point are mere temptations, as the gorge's most dramatic views are accessible only to hikers.

A 5-mile loop trail encircles much of the 3-mile gulf. Be aware that the trail lies directly along the gorge rim, and that the path is strewn with exposed tree roots, so take care at all times. Hikers can begin their trek on either the north or south rim. To obtain the best views, which are only accessible where the trails meet on the gorge's western end, plan to complete the entire circuit. The only significant difference between the two trails is that the South Rim Trail has

a watch tower that offers views to the east. On the eastern segment of the trails, the gorge's sides are steep but heavily vegetated. Consequently, views across the gulf offer only brief glimpses of the drastic erosion that has taken place. As hikers move west, the gorge narrows, the sides become more sheer, and the vegetation thins to reveal exposed shale. At the western end, the gulf's 385-foot walls are vertical and fully exposed. Campers visiting the park shouldn't miss these dramatic views.

Other activities and amenities within the park's boundaries include an exercise trail, as well as fishing and canoeing in the Whetstone Gulf Reservoir. The reservoir was constructed to provide flood control of Whetstone Creek, as well as recreational opportunities. Tiger muskies and largemouth bass stock the reservoir, which is accessible from Corrigan Hill Road.

Hikers wanting more-extensive trails can also visit the Lesser Wilderness State Forest, which borders much of Whetstone

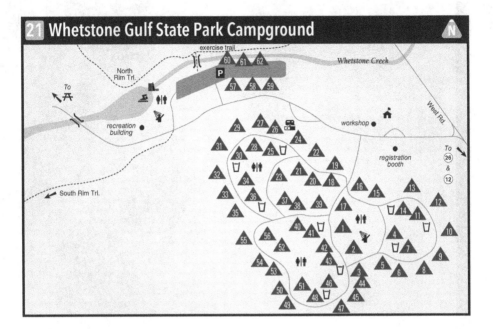

Gulf State Park. Whetstone's 2,100 acres, combined with Lesser Wilderness's 13,793, make for an extensive, continuous wilderness area. Hiking the access roads and trails, and fishing the streams and brooks, expand the outdoor recreational activities directly accessible from the park.

The Tug Hill area has many state forests, recreation areas, and wildlife-management areas with hiking, bicycling, fishing, canoeing, and kayaking opportunities—so travelers may want to consider Whetstone Gulf as a base camp to explore other points of interest in the Lesser Wilderness.

:: Getting There

From I-90 (New York State Thruway), take Exit 31, NY 8/NY 12. After toll, turn right on Genesee Street toward I-790 West/NY 5. Turn right on Aubert Avenue and merge onto I-790 West/NY 5 toward NY 12/NY 8. Merge onto NY 12 North toward Poland/Watertown, and follow it 29.5 miles. The park entrance is on the right.

GPS COORDINATES   N43° 42.150'   W75° 72.617'

Adirondacks

22

Adirondak Loj:
Wilderness Campground at Heart Lake

A perfectly situated backpacker's haven

Hikers, take note: the campground with the best real estate in the Adirondacks is not a DEC property. Nestled in the heart of the High Peaks, Adirondak Loj and the adjacent campground at Heart Lake are a perfectly situated backpacker's haven owned by the Adirondack Mountain Club (ADK). Since 1922, the ADK has been promoting a balance of "outdoor recreation, advocacy, environmental education, and natural resource conservation," according to its mission statement. As part of their mission, they operate a unique property with a variety of lodging experiences, from tent sites, lean-tos, and canvas cabins to a traditional cabin and rustic rooms within the historic Loj (which is to say nothing of the ADK's nearby hike-in properties: John Brooks Lodge, Grace Camp, and Camp Peggy O'Brien).

Of course, when we visit we usually opt for the tent sites or lean-tos. The rates may seem pricey compared with those of state campgrounds, but be aware that you won't be paying extra reservation fees to middlemen (ahem, ReserveAmerica). What you get for your extra cash is a base camp at the foot of New York's tallest mountains, a private swatch of sandy beach on picturesque Heart Lake, well-maintained facilities, a coveted parking spot, and easy access to the High Peaks Information Center. And as a bonus, you'll be supporting a great organization.

Though this campground has *wilderness* in its name and animals such as black bears visit frequently, don't let the wording fool you too much. While the lean-tos are hike-in, all of the tent sites are drive-in. The campground has the standard well-distributed drinking-water spigots and two comfort stations, including a small seasonal one available only to campers and a larger one at the High Peaks Information Center that's open to the public during regular business hours. The tent sites are situated along the edges of two loops, and while most are close to the road, they are all well spaced and nicely wooded with evergreens. You won't be able to reserve a particular site until you arrive and register, but among our favorites are numbers 23 and 24, which are tucked away at the end of their own private spurs. Unless the place is booked solid, we would avoid number 21, which sits in a small clearing next to the seasonal comfort station.

For even more privacy and a traditional Adirondack wilderness experience, sleep in a lean-to. These simple wooden structures have a sloping roof and are open to the elements on one side. On a nice, bug-free evening, the platform serves as a great place to unfurl your

:: Ratings

BEAUTY: ★ ★ ★ ★
PRIVACY: ★ ★ ★
QUIET: ★ ★ ★
CLEANLINESS: ★ ★ ★
SECURITY: ★ ★ ★ ★
SPACIOUSNESS: ★ ★ ★

:: Key Information

ADDRESS: 1002 Adirondak Loj Rd., Lake Placid, NY 12946

OPERATED BY: Adirondack Mountain Club

CONTACT: 518-523-3441; tinyurl.com/adkcampground

OPEN: Year-round

SITES: 32 tent sites and 16 lean-tos

SITE AMENITIES: Picnic table and fire ring

ASSIGNMENT: Choose from available sites

REGISTRATION: On arrival

FACILITIES: Water, pit and flush toilets, showers

PARKING: At site for tent sites, in lot for lean-tos; $5/day for additional vehicles

FEE: Tent site: $40/night May–October; $20/night November–April; lean-tos: $44/night May–October; $22/night November–April; all rates for 2 people, $5/night for each additional person; 10% off for Adirondack Mountain Club (ADK) members

ELEVATION: 1,657'

RESTRICTIONS:

■ **Pets:** Dogs on leash with proof of currently valid rabies vaccination

■ **Fires:** In fire rings only

■ **Alcohol:** At site

■ **Vehicles:** Up to 30'

■ **Other:** Quiet hours 10 p.m.–7 a.m.

■ **Reservations:** 1-night stay allowed

sleeping pad and bag, though if inclement weather arrives, you might wish you had your trusty nylon stand-by. Each of the lean-tos is found in the eastern half of the campground beyond the ring of tent sites. You will need to park in small lots and pack your gear in, but for no more than a few dozen yards. Choose from woodsy (sites 10–16) or water views (sites 1–9). Don't be fooled by the campground map. Sites 5–7 look as if they're waterfront, but in reality they are set back from the lake. The views, however, are still lovely. We would choose between site 8, with its lake view, and sites 2 and 3, with their secluded locale next to a small brook.

Recent additions to the campground are the canvas cabins, six permanent platform tents with bunk beds and mattresses. They're more expensive, but extremely convenient, especially if you have a big family. Just be warned that even on mildly windy nights, the walls of these "cabins" shudder and shake. For yet one more lodging alternative, book a

bed in the Adirondak Loj, built in 1927. This (relatively) luxe option comes complete with indoor plumbing, a meal plan in the dining room, and access to the Great Room with its inviting fireplace—just choose between private rooms, bunk rooms, or the hiker's loft.

Wherever you decide to rest your head, rise early to tackle the trail of your choice. Family-friendly Mount Jo loop offers beginners a nice place to start and requires minimal effort to reach views of Heart Lake and the campground. Day trips to Marcy Dam (where many thru-hikers spend the night) and on to Avalanche Pass serve up some spectacular vistas but don't require much climbing. Many hikers, however, use the Loj as the jumping-off point for two of the state's finest climbs: Mount Marcy and Algonquin Peak. At 5,334 feet, Marcy is the highest peak in the state and an essential check on any peak-bagging list, but be warned that the shortest round-trip from the campground is 15 miles, making for a long day. Algonquin is twice as

22 Adirondak Loj: Wilderness Campground at Heart Lake

close and 200 feet shorter, but it's a steeper scramble, and arguably prettier.

It's hard to ignore the popularity of the many trailheads at the campground, especially on busy summer weekends. Be grateful that if you book a site, you can simply walk from your sleeping bag to the trail register, rather than arriving before dawn and trying to secure one of the limited parking spaces. While summer (outside of black fly season) and fall are great times to visit, a cold-weather excursion can be beautiful in its own way, and it comes with lower rates and far fewer crowds. Many of the tent and lean-to sites operate year-round and the property is adjacent to an extensive cross-country trail system. Plus the High Peaks Information Center rents both cross-country skis and snowshoes. A trek out to see snow hugging the peaks at Avalanche Pass is one of the Adirondack's great adventures.

Still, we realize that not all campers are up for such extreme undertakings. Luckily, Lake Placid waits less than 10 miles away with its many restaurants, shops, and vacation amusements, not to mention its Olympic training center. Even closer to the campground, you can visit the farm of abolitionist John Brown, where he lived before his raid on Harpers Ferry. No matter when you come to pitch your tent, you will find a hike, an activity, or a tour to fill your day.

:: Getting There

From I-87 (Adirondack Northway), take Exit 30 to NY 73. Follow NY 73 for 26 miles and turn left onto Adirondak Loj Road at the sign for the High Peaks trailhead. Follow Adirondak Loj Road 5 miles to Heart Lake Center. The campground entrance will be directly ahead; check-in is at Adirondak Loj, to the right.

GPS COORDINATES   N44° 10.983'   W73° 57.833'

23

Alger Island

Enjoy private lakeside camping in the heart of the Adirondacks.

This scenic campground is located at the western end of Fourth Lake, a central part of the Fulton Chain of Lakes. The Fulton Chain is a series of connected lakes that begins at Old Forge Pond and ends at Eighth Lake. The first five lakes stretch unbroken for 14 miles. Old Forge Pond and Sixth through Eighth Lakes are separated from this main expanse by a series of channels. Steamboat inventor Robert Fulton envisioned connecting the lakes and creating an "Adirondack Canal." Although the canal was never built, the lakes still bear Fulton's name.

The lakes were eventually dammed and connected to provide flood control, recreational opportunities, and power in Lyons Falls. The shores are dotted with numerous summer "camps," or private residences, and boathouses—not mere storage buildings for boats, but actual homes ranging from quaint cottages to luxurious estates dating back to the Gilded Age. Though the shoreline is certainly developed, the area is heavily wooded. Views from the lakes reveal rocky outcrops and a vast, serene wilderness that have drawn outdoors enthusiasts to this region for generations.

:: Ratings

BEAUTY: ★ ★ ★ ★
PRIVACY: ★ ★ ★ ★
QUIET: ★ ★ ★
CLEANLINESS: ★ ★ ★ ★
SECURITY: ★ ★ ★ ★ ★
SPACIOUSNESS: ★ ★ ★

First known as Deer Island, then Big Island, Alger Island acquired its present name from its longtime owners, Mort and Ollie Alger. The state acquired the island in 1950 and began to build lean-tos in the 1960s. Each site is heavily wooded with evergreens and situated a stone's throw from the water's edge. Sites along the northern shore face the lakes' main channel, so boat tours, water-skiers, and Jet Skis are occasional disturbances during the day. A charming lighthouse is visible from the northern shore. Sites on the southern shore border a small inlet and provide more seclusion. Access is limited to registered campers, and isolation from the mainland ensures privacy and security.

Campers should be aware that the only way to get to the island is by boat. A state-owned boat launch is located at the Fourth Lake picnic area. This picnic area also serves as the Alger Island registration and permitting station. Boats launched at this facility are limited to car-top boats such as canoes and kayaks; motorboats can be launched from the public launch in Inlet. For campers who don't own boats, numerous outfitters along NY 28 not only rent boats but also offer rafting packages. This campground's popularity is evident; most sites are fully booked during July and August, with the most popular sites booked a year in advance.

Hiking at the campground is limited to a perimeter trail, but access to the West-Central region of the Adirondacks provides miles of hiking opportunities. Terrain in the region is generally hilly and rugged but

:: Key Information

ADDRESS: 303 Petrie Rd., Old Forge, NY 13420

OPERATED BY: New York State Department of Environmental Conservation

CONTACT: 315-369-3224; www.dec.ny.gov/outdoor/24451.html

OPEN: Mid-May–early September

SITES: 15 lean-to sites, 2 tent sites

SITE AMENITIES: Lean-to (except the 2 tent sites), pit toilet, and fire ring

ASSIGNMENT: Reservations

REGISTRATION: Noon–9 p.m.; required for access to island

FACILITIES: Picnic area, potable water, docks, lean-tos

PARKING: At Fourth Lake picnic area

FEE: $18/night

ELEVATION: 520'

RESTRICTIONS:

■ **Pets:** Dogs on leash with proof of currently valid rabies vaccination

■ **Fires:** In fire rings only

■ **Alcohol:** Allowed

■ **Vehicles:** None permitted; sites are accessible only by boat.

■ **Other:** Quiet hours 10 p.m.–7 a.m.; access only by boat

■ **Reservations:** None required for the 2 tent sites, required for lean-tos; 2-night stay required

not mountainous. Most of the surrounding area is heavily forested and within the protected New York Forest Preserve area of the Adirondack Park. Trails are often old logging roads that have become overgrown as they transform back into wilderness. Large, expansive views are limited, but numerous lakes, ponds, swamps, and streams present surprises around every corner. Most trails can be explored as day hikes and reached from NY 12 and NY 28. For in-depth descriptions of nearby trails, as well as hiking trails throughout the Adirondack region, see *Five-Star Trails in the Adirondacks* (Menasha Ridge Press, 2010).

Fishing is permitted at the campground and on the lake with a New York State fishing license. Smallmouth bass, lake trout, brook trout, rainbow trout, and landlocked Atlantic salmon call Fourth Lake home, and muskie and largemouth bass can be caught in some of the adjoining Fulton Chain of Lakes. You may swim in the lake but without a designated swimming area; swimmers should be mindful of boating activities nearby. A sandbar on the north shore near site 6 offers the best swimming area. Motorboats, canoes, and rowboats can be tied up at the docks on the southern or eastern shores; this allows campers to participate in a variety of Fulton Chain boating activities.

Considered the main tourist destination of the West-Central region, the town of Old Forge offers many attractions for those interested in local history and entertainment. Of note are the renovated theater, water park, Old Forge Hardware Store, and the Adirondack Scenic Railroad. You may purchase supplies and equipment along NY 28 from numerous outfitters, and also in small grocery stores in Old Forge, Eagle Bay, or Inlet.

Alger Island Campground's rocky shores and evergreen canopy provide a unique lakeside camping experience in one of New York's most cherished parks and wilderness areas. Outdoor activities abound in the region, and proximity to Old Forge allows campers to easily stock up on supplies and equipment.

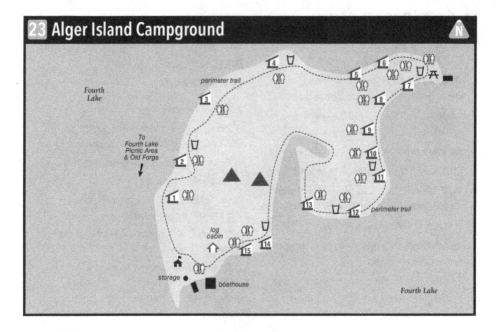

:: Getting There

Follow the directions for Whetstone Gulf State Park Campground (see page 79) through the fourth sentence, but take NY 12 North 22.3 miles. Bear right onto NY 28 North and drive 26.7 miles to Old Forge. Turn right on Gilbert Street, left on Park Avenue, and then right on South Shore Road. After 5.9 miles, make a sharp left onto Petrie Road. Fourth Lake Picnic Area is 0.75 mile ahead, on the left.

GPS COORDINATES (FOURTH LAKE PICNIC AREA)   N43° 44.150'   W74° 52.500'

GPS COORDINATES (ALGER ISLAND)   N43° 44.550'   W74° 52.617'

24

Ausable Point

It's a relatively young campground (built in 1965), but Ausable Point sits on the shores of a body of water with a long history.

As the Ausable River empties into Lake Champlain (the 100-plus-mile-long sliver of water that forms the northeastern border between New York and Vermont), it creates a fertile delta. Birds, and in turn birders, flock to these wetlands every spring and summer. The state has designated it the Ausable Marsh Wildlife Management Area, and with a keen eye and a good set of binoculars, you can spot ospreys, mergansers, teals, and goldeneyes within the 12 distinct ecological communities. Perhaps you will even spy a tent camper or two—because down the road, where the north branch of the Ausable meets the shores of Champlain, Ausable Point Campground houses 123 excellent campsites.

The campground entrance road leads along the northern border of Ausable Marsh. Even if you're not a birder, pull over and read the interpretive signs, or look out over the water from a viewing dock. A mile-long elevated foot trail will introduce you to some of the ecological communities, including emergent marsh, floodplain forest, and marsh headwater stream. If you do plan to

search for a bird or two, consult the excellent *Lake Champlain Birding Trail* brochure (**lakechamplainregion.com/recreation/outdoors/birding**) beforehand.

At the end of the road, just past the registration booth, is the campground's gem of a beach. More than a quarter-mile of sand makes up the large day-use area, complete with a relatively new pavilion and bathhouse. On summer days, lifeguards oversee the designated swimming areas. The size of the parking area testifies to the number of day visitors that use the beach and picnic area. Be prepared to share. The silver lining: no vendors hawk pizza and fried food, and that helps keep some folks away. East of the beach is a separate windsurfing area known as the Stone Jetty. If the crowds at the swimming beach are a bit too oppressive, drop your beach chair near the jetty and enjoy the sight of windsurfers and boaters gliding along Lake Champlain's waters past the heavily wooded backdrop of Valcour Island.

Just south of Stone Jetty, you'll find the relatively private, grass-and-sand campsites. They are laid out in four separate loops, each with its own comfort station and multiple sources of running water. Sites 1–24 are closest to the jetty—and with the windsurfer loading area, the camp's shower building, and a swing set all nearby, this loop tends to be the noisiest during the day. But it also contains the most sites on the edge of Lake Champlain, including 9, 10, 11, 13, 15, 16, 19, 20, 21, and 22.

:: Ratings

BEAUTY: ★ ★ ★
PRIVACY: ★ ★
QUIET: ★ ★ ★
CLEANLINESS: ★ ★ ★
SECURITY: ★ ★ ★
SPACIOUSNESS: ★ ★ ★

:: Key Information

ADDRESS: 3346 Lake Shore Rd., Peru, NY 12972	**FACILITIES:** Water, flush toilets, showers
OPERATED BY: New York State Department of Environmental Conservation	**PARKING:** At site; maximum 2 vehicles
	FEE: $22/night
CONTACT: 518-561-7080; www.dec.ny.gov/outdoor/24452.html	**ELEVATION:** 98'
OPEN: Mid-May–early October	**RESTRICTIONS:**
SITES: 123	▓ **Pets:** Dogs on leash with proof of currently valid rabies vaccination
SITE AMENITIES: Picnic table and fire ring	▓ **Fires:** In fire rings only
ASSIGNMENT: Choose from available sites or reservations	▓ **Alcohol:** At site
	▓ **Vehicles:** Up to 45'
REGISTRATION: On arrival or by reservation	▓ **Other:** Quiet hours 10 p.m.–7 a.m.
	▓ **Reservations:** 2-night stay required

These sites, separated by privacy hedges, are usually booked far in advance. However, we found the second loop (25–48 and 81–83) just as desirable. Sites on the eastern perimeter of the loop border a small, grassy marsh. The North Branch of the Ausable skirts the edge of the southern sites. The spacious site 27 was a favorite, ideal for a larger group. Site 28 is sandy and opens onto a small beach—but don't forget that wading and swimming are allowed only at the lifeguard beach.

If you are looking for less through-traffic, consider sites 49–80, but be warned that the foliage in this section does not provide as much privacy as one would hope. A small path between sites 77 and 78 takes you directly to the beach, and this may appeal to families with little ones.

Sites 84–123 used to be the favorites for RVs, but not anymore. They pulled the plug on these former electric sites in the winter of 2006 because of safety concerns and requirements to keep Adirondack campgrounds rustic. This change has certainly lowered the number of RVs visiting the campground and shortened the length of some visits, but generators can still be heard during designated hours. Try to avoid these sites in the spring or after a storm. With the Ausable running nearby, this section of the campground tends to flood.

Lake Champlain's wide waters are suitable for boats of all types. Paddling is best close to shore, and the only launch in the campground is for car-top boats. You'll find a public trailer launch 3 miles away at the Peru Docks. Anglers try to catch bass, trout, salmon, bullhead perch, walleye, carp, smelt, eel, crappie, or bluegill from boats or the shore.

It's a relatively young campground (built in 1965), but Ausable Point sits on the shores of a body of water with a long human history. American Indians first settled in the lake's valley more than 10,000 years ago. Samuel de Champlain, the European who inspired the lake's current name, first sailed these waters in 1609. For a great tribute to Champlain, check out Crown Point, about an hour's drive to the south. Historic forts and the Champlain Memorial Lighthouse make it worth a stop.

24 Ausable Point Campground

West of the lake, just minutes from the campground, the Ausable River thunders through a narrow gorge for 2 miles, forming Ausable Chasm. Sometimes called Little Grand Canyon of the East, this is not to be confused with the Grand Canyon of the East in Letchworth State Park (see page 172). Day-trippers can use the free parking lot, walk over the chasm bridge, and take in the spectacular waterfall and the churning waters that stand in stark contrast to the placid delta where the river empties into Lake Champlain.

:: Getting There

From I-87 (Adirondack Northway), take Exit 35 to CR 442. Follow CR 442 for 2 miles and turn left on NY 9 North. Drive 0.5 mile to the campground entrance, on the right.

GPS COORDINATES   N44° 34.783'   W73° 26.483'

25

Brown Tract Pond

Tucked away from the main tourist areas of Adirondack Park is the 146-acre Brown Tract Pond, whose rugged shores offer tent campers a quiet wilderness setting.

Say the word *Adirondacks*, and most people envision placid bodies of water with forested and boulder-strewn shores—the very picture of a tranquil wilderness. During the tourist season, campers who seek these settings usually have to hike or boat to primitive campsites—but the Brown Tract Pond campground offers such opportunities for the car camper. Tucked away from the main tourist areas of the Adirondack Park is the 146-acre Brown Tract Pond, whose rugged shores offer tent campers a quiet wilderness setting. Power boats are not allowed on the pond—and given the remote setting, the loudest sounds you are likely to hear will be the calls of a loon.

The campground consists of three separate areas—one neighboring the entrance, one past the day-use area, and one along Uncas Road. The first area includes sites 1–37, though the numbering does not follow the direction of travel through the area. The first few grassy sites (30–32) are relatively open, with some shade provided by evergreens that obscure views of the pond. As you drive up a small hill, the canopy of evergreens closes, shading the area more thoroughly. Clustered together along the hill are sites 22–29, all of which lie on the pond side of the road and have views of the water. Campers should note that sites 23 and 26 are walk-in sites, but because they are directly on the shore, they are very desirable.

Across the road and near the area's comfort station are sites 20 and 21, which are similar to the previous sites but lack views of the pond. Atop the hill, undergrowth is notably absent due to the thickening of the evergreen canopy, but campers who prefer views over privacy would be well suited to the pond side of the road, as the views here are expansive. Across the road, the sites begin to blend into the mixed-hardwood forest, offering some privacy at the expense of views of the pond. The one-way route out of the area dips into a small hollow that contains sites 1–6. Shaded by hardwoods and surrounded by vegetation, these sites feel more private but none have views of the water and all are smaller than previous sites.

The last few sites (33–37) in the area lie on a separate road next to the pond and are surrounded by thick brush. Though tall shade trees are notably absent from this area, these sites are deep and private. Given the beautiful views of the pond, these sites are definitely among the top choices.

:: Ratings

BEAUTY: ★ ★ ★ ★ ★
PRIVACY: ★ ★ ★ ★
QUIET: ★ ★ ★ ★ ★
CLEANLINESS: ★ ★ ★ ★
SECURITY: ★ ★ ★ ★
SPACIOUSNESS: ★ ★ ★

:: Key Information

ADDRESS: Uncas Road,
Raquette Lake, NY 13436

OPERATED BY: New York State Department of Environmental Conservation

CONTACT: 315-354-4412; www.dec.ny
.gov/outdoor/24456.html

OPEN: Mid-May–Labor Day

SITES: 90 tent sites

SITE AMENITIES: Picnic table and
fire ring

ASSIGNMENT: Choose from available
sites or reservations

REGISTRATION: Noon–9 p.m.

FACILITIES: Picnic areas, potable water,
flush toilets, boat launch and rentals

PARKING: At site

FEE: $18/night

ELEVATION: 1,788'

RESTRICTIONS:

■ **Pets:** Dogs on leash with proof of
currently valid rabies vaccination

■ **Fires:** In fire rings only

■ **Alcohol:** Allowed

■ **Vehicles:** RVs and trailers allowed

■ **Other:** Quiet hours 10 p.m.–7 a.m.;
no motorboats allowed

■ **Reservations:** 2-night stay required

The next camping area is past an evergreen swamp and the public picnic area. The first few sites (38, 48, and 49) sit at a crossroads and are consequently fairly public. The road forks at this point: right is a steep climb to sites 50–81; left is to the boat launch and sites 39–47. Sites on the left fork hug the pond's shore (except for site 41), and all have excellent views of the water. Short hardwoods provide intermittent shade, but there is little vegetation in the area to provide real seclusion.

As you bear right and drive up the steep hill, the character of the campground changes, as tall hardwoods predominate and a dense woodland feel pervades the area. Sites 50 and 51 along the steep climb are very deep and spacious. Atop the hill are two large, grassy, open sites (52 and 53), after which the road forks to form a loop. Near this fork are short driveways for the walk-in sites (55, 56, and 58) that are situated among rugged woodlands—this creates a remote feel but leaves little room to spread out. The central sites and upper part of the loop are generally

encircled by a dense understory, which creates smaller but isolated sites. At the back of the loop, a short spur road provides access to some rustic and interesting sites: 68–70. Sites 69 and 70 are walk-in; because they sit high above the water, they offer interesting views of the pond and the surrounding wilderness, particularly site 70. The dense woodland and rugged terrain create sites that are wonderfully secluded from the rest of the campground but not so secluded from each other, being clustered close together. The next four sites (71–74) share access, and although 73 is a secluded walk-in site similar to 69 and 70, the other sites in this group huddle around a sandy drive. The rest of the sites along the perimeter of this loop are secluded and well forested, with good views of the pond. The last three sites, 80–82, are short walk-ins down the hill; these woodland sites afford plenty of privacy.

Access to the last camping area is directly off Uncas Road; consequently, the sites here are removed from the rest of the campground. The large and spacious

25 Brown Tract Pond Campground

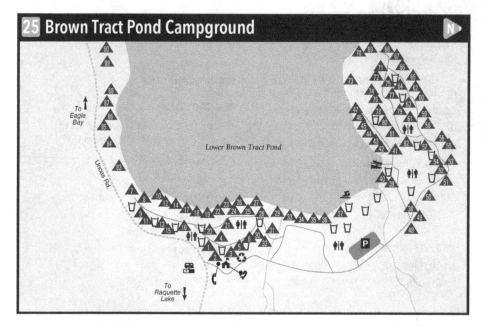

sites are heavily wooded and offer great views of the pond. The area does not have a comfort station but rather is served by pit toilets. Their proximity to a public dirt road may raise security issues for some campers, but considering the remote location of the campground and the lack of traffic on the bumpy road, this issue is easily overlooked. Indeed, these sites are the first to fill up, and because they offer a private lakeside setting, it is certainly worth taking a look to see what is available.

:: Getting There

Follow the directions for Alger Island Campground (see page 86) through the first sentence. Bear right onto NY 28 North, but drive 11.3 miles past Old Forge and Inlet to Raquette Lake Village. Turn left on CR 2; go 0.5 mile past the general store (CR 2 becomes Antlers Road). After 0.2 mile, turn left on Uncas Road. The campground entrance is 1.8 miles ahead, on the right.

GPS COORDINATES   N43° 48.633'   W74° 41.683'

26

Buck Pond

Buck Pond is a haven for paddlers.

More than 20 miles north of Lake Placid and less than 50 miles south of Quebec, Buck Pond is a truly remote campground and one of our favorites in the Adirondacks. Visitors to the region, including many Canadians, do not come here to find antiques or stay at scenic inns. They come for the woods and the water, and Buck Pond is a haven for paddlers.

Situated between Buck Pond on the east, Kushaqua Narrows on the west, and Lake Kushaqua on the north, the campground is surrounded by water. During the summer, most campers (a mix of RVs, pop-ups, and tents) are likely to have at least one boat with them. If you cannot bring your own, there are canoes and rowboats to rent and local outfitters to load you up with gear.

Regulations vary on each body of water. No motorboats are allowed on Buck Pond, guaranteeing a quieter scene. Campers slide their canoes and kayaks into the water from the car-top boat launch. Lake Kushaqua and its trailer boat launch offer opportunities for larger (and faster) vessels. Paddlers can travel 7 continuous miles in the water, or more than 100 miles to Old Forge if they don't mind a handful of portages. Less ambitious? If you can carry your boat three-quarters of a mile, a float to the village of Paul Smiths (about 10 miles away by car) is possible. Canoeists and kayakers alike enjoy this trip through the Kushaqua Narrows, Rainbow Lake, Jones Pond, and Osgood Pond. Or continue south from Paul Smiths to Saranac Lakes, or west into the "forever wild" waters of the St. Regis Canoe Area. Just plan ahead and, as the campground brochure suggests, have a car waiting at the other end.

Anglers enjoy visits to the campground, as well. They pull up brown bullhead, northern pike, and yellow perch from Buck Pond and black bass and rainbow trout from Lake Kushaqua. Up the road near Mud Pond, the North Branch of the Saranac River is a good place to find brook trout. If you are turned off by the name Mud Pond, consider that countless bodies of water in the Adirondacks bear this uninviting moniker. As the story goes, some of the best fishing spots are near or on "Mud Ponds," and they were so named to dissuade everyone except for locals.

Come to think of it, "Buck Pond" isn't the nicest of names either, but the campground is certainly a fine one. Driving along the camp road (formerly the route of the Delaware & Hudson railbed), you may notice the subtle design details that increase one's sense of privacy. The sites are thick with mixed hardwoods and a full understory that shelters campers from their neighbors and the sun. But the angled entrances and

:: Ratings

BEAUTY: ★ ★ ★ ★
PRIVACY: ★ ★ ★ ★
QUIET: ★ ★ ★ ★
CLEANLINESS: ★ ★ ★ ★
SECURITY: ★ ★ ★ ★
SPACIOUSNESS: ★ ★ ★ ★

:: Key Information

ADDRESS: CR 60, P.O. Box 9A, Onchiota, NY 12989

OPERATED BY: New York State Department of Environmental Conservation

CONTACT: 518-891-3449; www.dec.ny .gov/outdoor/24457.html

OPEN: Mid-May–early September

SITES: 116

SITE AMENITIES: Picnic table and fire ring

ASSIGNMENT: Choose from available sites or reservations

REGISTRATION: On arrival or by reservation

FACILITIES: Water, pit and flush toilets, showers

PARKING: At site, maximum 2 vehicles

FEE: $20/night

ELEVATION: 1,696'

RESTRICTIONS:

■ **Pets:** Dogs on leash with proof of currently valid rabies vaccination

■ **Fires:** In fire rings only

■ **Alcohol:** At site

■ **Vehicles:** Up to 30'

■ **Other:** Quiet hours 10 p.m.–7 a.m.; motorboats allowed on Lake Kushaqua but prohibited on Buck Pond

■ **Reservations:** 1-night stay allowed

staggered sites make the biggest difference. Views of campers from one site to another are rare. If only more campgrounds were this well planned. Another nice touch: each comfort station includes at least one shower, so there's no need for a long walk (or drive) to a common bathhouse.

Loops A and B curl off to the right just past the registration booth. Sites in Loop A fill up quickly, especially those nearest the water (9, 12, 13, 15, 17, 19, 20, and 21). Along the edge of the campground in Loop B, site 56 is a good choice for those who want even more privacy. Loop C, a double loop with rougher roads, includes some of the sites closest to Lake Kushaqua (most notably sites 89, 91, 92, and 94). It's hard to go wrong with any sites in the campground, though. Even the seven sites in tiny Loop D, near the recycling center, are well spread out.

By far, the most desired are two boat-access sites that are usually booked solid months in advance. A literal stone's throw across the water from 91 and 92, sites R-1 and R-2 sit on a small island and feature the standard fire ring and picnic table, along with pit toilets. Campers could probably wade over to the island, but it is still a nice thought to be sharing your land with just one other group. Even if you do not get an island site, relax at the sandy bathing beach and take in the impressive views of Big Haystack and Kate Mountains.

Hiking is obviously another attraction, with a popular short trail following the former railbed. It's a little more than a mile to the outlet of Lake Kushaqua. For those looking to venture farther from camp, St. Regis Mountain in Paul Smiths and Debar Mountain at Meacham Lake are known for expansive vistas. Another option is the short but steep trail up Little Haystack. Be careful, though. The trail is not very well marked.

One of the great things about the Adirondacks is its tradition of wilderness guides. For almost 200 years, these men and women have outfitted and led groups on trips in the woods, on the water, or both. Today,

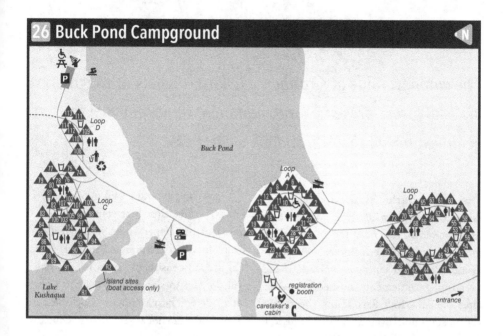

26 Buck Pond Campground

modern conveniences and technology make the wilderness more accessible to all, but that does not make it any less dangerous. Hiring an Adirondack guide is a great way to introduce yourself safely to a new area. When we visited Buck Pond, the caretaker informed us that he was a licensed guide. It was pleasant to see a business card that summarizes one's offerings as "Fishing, Paddling, Photography, and Snowshoeing."

:: Getting There

From I-87 (Adirondack Northway), take Exit 30 to NY 73 North. Follow NY 73 North for 28 miles. In Lake Placid, take NY 86 West for 9 miles into the village of Saranac Lake. Turn right on NY 3 East. After 6.5 miles, continue onto State Street/Oregon Plains Road. After 6 miles, turn right on CR 60/Gabriels–Onchiota Road and follow it 1.5 miles to the campground entrance, on your left.

GPS COORDINATES   N44° 29.750'   W74° 07.033'

27

Cranberry Lake

The campgrounds at Cranberry Lake are adjacent to 150,000 acres of forest-preserve land, making it an ideal place to begin exploring the Adirondack wilderness.

The Adirondacks' rugged terrain and dense woodlands made most of the area inhospitable for American Indians as well as for early settlers. The region served mostly as a battleground during colonization, and as farming settlements pushed westward after the American Revolution, the region lay mostly undiscovered. As the Industrial Age came into full swing, the region was exploited heavily for timber and minerals, but along with this exploitation came the region's first vacationers. Following their arrival, a growing acceptance of the inherent value of wilderness, along with recognition of the devastation wrought by the demands of industry in the area, created a movement to preserve the remaining wilderness. Consequently, the Adirondack Park and Forest Preserve was created to preserve these lands. The campgrounds at Cranberry Lake are adjacent to 150,000 acres of forest-preserve land, making it an ideal place to begin exploring the Adirondack wilderness.

:: Ratings

BEAUTY: ★ ★ ★ ★
PRIVACY: ★ ★ ★
QUIET: ★ ★ ★ ★
CLEANLINESS: ★ ★ ★
SECURITY: ★ ★ ★ ★
SPACIOUSNESS: ★ ★ ★

The campground is laid out in two sections. The first, close to the entrance, is composed of the Upper Loop, Roadside Loop, Bear Mountain Loop, and Peninsula Loop. The second consists of Loops I–V. Campers will do best to skip sites along the Upper, Roadside, and Bear Mountain Loops, because the majority are not as secluded, spacious, or scenic as sites along the other loops.

The Peninsula Loop sites (31–55) are well spaced, sit back from the road, and are surrounded by thick saplings, ferns, and other woodland vegetation. The southern part of the loop is adjacent to the lake, which becomes visible near site 40. A spur road with a tight turnaround heads left at this point, bringing you to sites 41–45. These sites hug the turnaround but have excellent views out to the lake. Complementing the views, the sites are larger than those encountered so far, but the canopy thins along the shore, so there is less brush between sites. Expansive views are also available from sites 46–48, but as the loop turns back toward the main road, they diminish. However, the undergrowth thickens and the sites become even larger as you leave the loop.

A short drive south past the amphitheater and recycling and dump stations brings campers to Loops I–V. Although the dense canopy of hardwoods remains, the brush between sites thins. Large boulders and a

:: Key Information

ADDRESS: 243 Lone Pine Rd., Cranberry Lake, NY 12927

OPERATED BY: New York State Department of Environmental Conservation

CONTACT: 315-848-2315; www.dec.ny.gov/outdoor/24460.html

OPEN: Mid-May–mid-October

SITES: 173 tent sites

SITE AMENITIES: Picnic table and fire ring

ASSIGNMENT: Choose from available sites or reservations

REGISTRATION: 8 a.m.–9 p.m.

FACILITIES: Picnic areas, amphitheater, pavilion, potable water, flush toilets, swimming beach, bathhouse, showers

PARKING: At site

FEE: $20/night most tent sites

ELEVATION: 1,547'

RESTRICTIONS:

■ **Pets:** Dogs on leash with proof of currently valid rabies vaccination

■ **Fires:** In fire rings only

■ **Alcohol:** Allowed

■ **Vehicles:** RVs and trailers limited to specific sites

■ **Other:** Quiet hours 10 p.m.–7 a.m.

■ **Reservations:** 2-night stay required

plethora of ferns dot the area, enhancing the wilderness setting. In general, the central sites are smaller and closer together than those on the perimeter along Loops I–III. Additionally, the first and last sites along these loops are near the main road, so they are also smaller and less desirable. Obviously, the best sites have views of the lake—along Loop I, these include sites 61–69. The sites on the perimeter here blend in with the rocky shore of the lake, providing picturesque campsites. Along Loop II, the sites with views of the lake begin at site 88 and end near site 98. Most sites along this loop are bigger than those described so far and will satisfy campers who desire more room. Loop III is elevated above its neighboring loops, and, consequently, partial views of the lake are present throughout. But the best lake views are from sites 117–124, because a tiny bay to the east partially surrounds these sites with water.

Loop IV essentially acts as the turnaround for the main road, so throughtraffic is a minor concern here. The sites, however, are spacious, deep, and more spread out than in previous loops. Campers who prize space and solitude should look here, as the area is definitely less crowded with sites, and the feel of a deep woodland is pervasive. Loop V continues this remote wilderness setting but with less effect, as there are more sites and a small interior loop that brings central sites closer to each other and the main road.

Directly east of the campground is Bear Mountain, which can be reached by several trails. As you could guess, one trailhead is on the Bear Mountain Loop, and another is on Loop IV. From atop Bear Mountain, hikers can look out upon Cranberry Lake and the vast forest preserves that await wilderness hikers. The Cranberry Lake Wild Forest, which surrounds the campground to the east and the lake to the west, has miles of hiking directly accessible from the campground. In addition, the Five Ponds Wilderness Area envelops the lake's southern shore and stretches miles to the west. Dozens of long trails can be reached from trailheads along CR 3 and adjoining roads.

:: Getting There

From I-81 North, take Exit 45, NY 3/Sackets Harbor/Downtown. Turn right on NY 3 and drive a little more than 70 miles to Cranberry Lake Village. Turn right on Lone Pine Road and continue a little more than a mile to the park entrance.

GPS COORDINATES   N44° 11.917'   W74° 49.550'

28

Eighth Lake

Views of the undeveloped and forested shores are exceptional —during the fall season they are emblazoned with color.

When visitors come to the Adirondacks, they are usually impressed with the sheer number of rugged hiking trails that crisscross the wilderness. One of the other ways to explore this vast wilderness—which often escapes first-time visitors—is the numerous canoe routes. Interconnected rivers, streams, ponds, and lakes provide innumerable miles of adventure; and when connected by short portages, the distances canoes can travel are truly vast. Although the rivers and rapids in the Adirondacks should only be attempted by experienced boaters or with an outfitter, the placid lakes and ponds are within grasp of most novice boaters. Indeed, one of the more easily navigable canoe trips in the western Adirondacks is along the Fulton Chain of Lakes. Roughly 20 miles long, part of this chain contains Seventh and Eighth Lakes—the second and third largest as well as the least developed. Nestled between these two lakes is Eighth Lake Campground.

The campground is actually divided into three separate areas: one on the shores of Eighth Lake, one on the shores of Seventh

Lake, and one (with a large number of sites) along the road between these areas. To access the sites along Eighth Lake's shore, drive past sites 1–9 (wooded and perfectly pleasant). Shaded by a mixture of pines and hardwoods, these sites have staggered drives and undergrowth for privacy. The next group of sites (11–20A) lies on an open lawn—although they back up to the woods, the woodland feel pervasive elsewhere in the campground is notably absent here. After passing these sites you have a choice: turn left and head to a group of sites within the shade of some very large pines (sites 46–54); or turn right along the lakeshore where the canopy becomes denser (sites 21–45). To the left, the tightly clustered group of sites is barely separated from the day-use area by a log fence, making them very public and not the choice for anyone seeking privacy.

Sites along the right fork and along the lakeshore side of the road are the real gems here and certainly the top choice of all the sites. Neighboring the boat launch for Eighth Lake, the first two sites (21 and 22) are more public than sites farther along the road. All the sites here are shaded by a mixture of hardwoods and softwoods, with lots of saplings and brush between. This, combined with ample space between sites, makes them ideal for campers seeking seclusion. Although sites across the road from the lake are nice woodland sites and offer glimpses of the lake, you can't beat the panoramic lake

:: Ratings

BEAUTY: ★ ★ ★ ★
PRIVACY: ★ ★ ★ ★
QUIET: ★ ★ ★ ★
CLEANLINESS: ★ ★ ★
SECURITY: ★ ★ ★
SPACIOUSNESS: ★ ★ ★ ★

:: Key Information

ADDRESS: 1353 NY 28, Inlet, NY 13360

OPERATED BY: New York State Department of Environmental Conservation

CONTACT: 315-345-4120; www.dec.ny .gov/outdoor/24465.html

OPEN: Mid-May–Columbus Day

SITES: 126 tent sites

SITE AMENITIES: Picnic table and fire ring

ASSIGNMENT: Choose from available sites or reservations

REGISTRATION: 3 p.m.–9 p.m.

FACILITIES: Picnic areas, swimming

beach, potable water, flush toilets, boat launch, showers

PARKING: At site

FEE: $22/night most tent sites

ELEVATION: 1,813'

RESTRICTIONS:

▓ **Pets:** Dogs on leash with proof of currently valid rabies vaccination

▓ **Fires:** In fire rings only

▓ **Alcohol:** Allowed

▓ **Vehicles:** RVs and trailers allowed

▓ **Other:** Quiet hours 10 p.m.–7 a.m.

▓ **Reservations:** 2-night stay required

views seen from the shore. A thin belt of small hemlocks and other saplings encompasses the lakeside sites from the shore, but a short walk through this band of saplings takes campers directly to the lake. A narrow, sandy beach stretches along the shore to site 37, beyond which grasses and stones take over. Views of the undeveloped and forested shores are exceptional—during the fall season they are emblazoned with color.

The 1-mile-long road south to Seventh Lake (which is also the canoe portage between the two lakes) contains more than 40 woodland sites. In fact, the Northern Forest Canoe Trail, which connects the Fulton Chain of Lakes to the northern tip of Maine via a 740-mile route through Vermont, Quebec, and New Hampshire, uses this road as a portage. Sites along this road blend into the forest, which transitions from dense pines along the western edge (found close to sites 55–68) to the more typical mixed-hardwood forest of the Adirondacks. All the sites in this

area are large and well distributed along the road, and staggered drives help keep the area private despite a thin understory. Although most sites here sit close to the road, they become deeper as you approach the loop near Seventh Lake.

The sites maintain the deep woodland feel of the portage road until near site 110, where views of Seventh Lake add a new depth to the wilderness setting. From sites 110–119, all of the sites have good views of the lake and a small, rugged island; at site 120, thick vegetation blocks the view. Generally the sites are a bit smaller here than elsewhere in the campground, but thicker brush enhances their privacy. Although all of the lakeside sites in this loop are close to the water and have magnificent views, of particular interest are sites 112 and 113, which are right on the water's edge. Note that the boat launch on this lake is close to sites 114A and 116, and don't forget to wave to the boaters on their way to Maine.

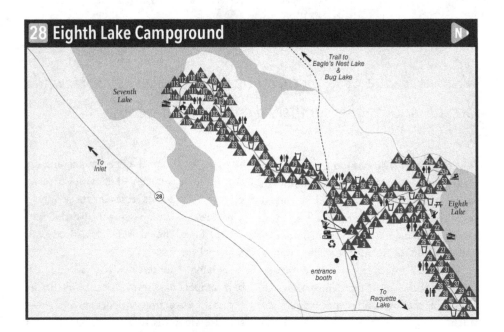

:: Getting There

Follow the directions for Alger Island Campground (see page 86) through the first sentence. Bear right onto NY 28 North and follow it 11.3 miles through Old Forge and Inlet. Continue along NY 28 North another 6.7 miles. The campground entrance is on your left.

GPS COORDINATES   N43° 45.950'   W74° 42.300'

29

Forked Lake

With views due west, picturesque sunsets over the water and forested shores give campers a special treat here.

Tent campers who seek the solitude and beauty of the wilderness could hardly go wrong visiting the campground at Forked Lake. The rocky, 1,248-acre lake is an ideal boating and fishing spot, though motorboats will find navigating the shallow waters in North Bay treacherous. Indeed, scrape marks on numerous concealed rocks reveal that even shallow-draft canoes often get caught along the shores. Most approaches to sites' landings or docks are littered with these concealed rocks, warranting a slow pace and cautious eye. Since it is doubtful that boaters would wish to subject their propellers and deeper hulls to these numerous hazards, and the trails between sites are rugged, canoes or kayaks seem the more practical means of getting around the bay and campground in general. Fortunately, campers who don't own a boat can rent canoes right off a rack next to the boat launch.

The sites on Forked Lake are essentially boat-only sites, though the majority of them can be accessed along footpaths (3–34 and 63–76). A few sites (1, 2, and 76–79) lie on

:: Ratings

BEAUTY: ★ ★ ★ ★ ★
PRIVACY: ★ ★ ★ ★ ★
QUIET: ★ ★ ★ ★ ★
CLEANLINESS: ★ ★ ★ ★ ★
SECURITY: ★ ★ ★ ★
SPACIOUSNESS: ★ ★ ★ ★

an open lawn near the boat launch and are accessible to vehicles—but with so many other excellent sites, consider these only as a last resort. Encompassing the North Bay of Forked Lake, the lakeside sites afford phenomenal views.

Going counterclockwise around the bay, campers pass several sites (3–7) that lie across the water from the boat launch. These sites are widely distributed among pines and short cedars, which seem to grow out of the rock-covered shores. For campers who don't have a boat or choose not to rent one, these will be the easiest sites to get to. Beyond site 7, the lake widens and you pass out of the visible range of the caretaker's cabin and any other vestiges of civilization.

Along these rugged shores, the sites (8–15) become even more spread out as they continue west and then wrap around a large rocky corner, where the sites sit higher above the lake. As the lakeshore turns nearly due north, the remaining sites (16–34) along the footpath become a little closer together. The sites are surrounded by tall pines and cedars, scrub, and an occasional hardwood extending its branches over the mostly open sites. These sites feel completely secluded, and there is plenty of room to set up. With views due west, picturesque sunsets over the water and forested shores give campers a special treat here.

The first boat-only site (35) is also on the eastern shore but is separated from the

:: Key Information

ADDRESS: 381 Forked Lake Campsite Ln., Long Lake, NY 12847

OPERATED BY: New York State Department of Environmental Conservation

CONTACT: 518-624-6646; www.dec.ny .gov/outdoor/24467.html

OPEN: Mid-May-Labor Day

SITES: 80 tent sites

SITE AMENITIES: Fire ring and bear box

ASSIGNMENT: Choose from available sites or reservations

REGISTRATION: Noon-9 p.m.

FACILITIES: Pit toilets, boat launch and rentals

PARKING: Near the boat launch

FEE: $18/night most tent sites

ELEVATION: 1,755'

RESTRICTIONS:

▇ **Pets:** Dogs on leash with proof of currently valid rabies vaccination

▇ **Fires:** In fire rings only

▇ **Alcohol:** Allowed

▇ **Vehicles:** RVs and trailers limited to specific sites

▇ **Other:** Quiet hours 10 p.m.-7 a.m.; food must be stored in food lockers

▇ **Reservations:** 2-night stay required

footpath sites by a marshy area and a small stream. This huge site is neighbored on its west by a larger stream, and the bay in front is covered by lily pads. Past the thick spread of lily pads, the boat-only sites mix in with dense evergreens and moss-covered boulders along the rock-covered shores. Widely spaced along the western shore, sites 36–49 are spacious and secluded. Site 39 is particularly isolated—it's at the tip of the mainland between a lily-pad bay to the north and a boulder-strewn bay to the south. The sunrise over distant mountains illuminates these sites, so early risers enjoy a wonderful scene out of their tent door.

Those who cannot decide between stunning sunrises or majestic sunsets could pick one of the island sites (50–52) and get both. Site 50 has its own private, forested, rocky island, whereas sites 51 and 52 share a slightly larger tree-covered island.

Past the islands and along a narrower strip of water, where the lake snakes west into Plumley Bay, are the last few boat-only sites (53–62). Dense pines shade these shores, and although the sites are not as spacious or spread out as some of the others, no sites here drop below a rating of "very desirable." Around the point and facing Plumley Bay are sites 60–62: if it is possible to feel more remote within this campground, these sites will do the trick.

A footpath serves the last remaining sites, which sit along the southern shore toward the boat launch and past the two islands. Evergreens grow tall here, making these forested sites the shadiest in the campground. With 12 sites spread over three-quarters of a mile, it's safe to assume you are guaranteed a private camping experience. Unique among these sites is site 75—large and grassy, with a sandy beach that faces west.

The only disclaimer for these wonderful sites is that they truly are primitive, so visitors should be mindful of their impact on the area. Pit toilets are the only facilities available, and the bear boxes for food storage at each site clearly indicate the need for conscientious food and trash management. And

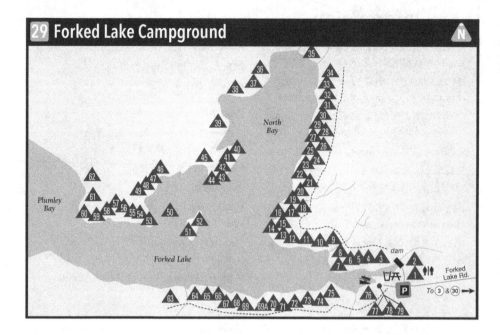

29 Forked Lake Campground

because access to the sites is very limited, campground staff relies on strict compliance with its carry-in/carry-out policy to ensure that the sites remain in their pristine state.

:: Getting There

Follow the directions for Alger Island Campground (see page 86) through the first sentence. Bear right onto NY 28 North and follow it 11.3 miles past Old Forge and Inlet; continue 23.7 miles. In Blue Mountain Lake, go straight on NY 28 North/ NY 30 for 7.5 miles. Go left on CR 3. Go nearly 3 miles; at the fork in road, bear right on Forked Lake Road. The campground entrance is 1.8 miles ahead.

GPS COORDINATES N43° 54.317' W74° 31.567'

30

Indian Lake Islands

If you have a tent and a boat, Indian Lake is the place to camp in the region.

In the central Adirondacks, equidistant between the towns of Speculator and Indian Lake, are two distinct campgrounds. The first is Lewey Lake, a group of sites located on or near the lake's 90 acres of water. The second is Indian Lake Islands, which is so close to Lewey that its entrance is located between Lewey's sites 35 and 37. The two offer very different camping experiences. Whereas Lewey offers a beach, the standard amenities, and many waterfront sites among its 209, it can be congested and lacks the beauty of many other campgrounds in the mountains. Conversely, Indian Lake Islands has only 55 sites on its 4,000 acres, all with boat-only access, offering unparalleled privacy and amazing views. If you have a tent and a boat, Indian Lake is the place to camp in the region. Even if you don't have a boat, canoes and kayaks are available to rent from the Department of Environmental Conservation (DEC) at the boat launch, and motorboats can be rented and delivered by marinas such as Dunn's Boat Service at Big Moose Lake. It would be hard to find an excuse not to visit.

:: Ratings

BEAUTY: ★ ★ ★ ★ ★
PRIVACY: ★ ★ ★ ★ ★
QUIET: ★ ★ ★ ★
CLEANLINESS: ★ ★ ★ ★
SECURITY: ★ ★ ★ ★
SPACIOUSNESS: ★ ★ ★ ★ ★

Indian Lake is long and narrow, with more than 7 miles of water stretching between sites 1 and 51. At the southern end are three forks, the westernmost leading to Lewey Lake and the campground entrance. Development on the lake is concentrated on the northern end in the town of Sabael, where the rustic Timberlock family resort and a smattering of vacation homes line the water. Campers, however, will find the lake is rarely crowded, and the well-spaced sites are all solitary retreats unto themselves. To even reach the main section of sites, it is a 2.5-mile paddle from the registration booth.

Among the islands, five of the smaller ones house single sites and are perennially popular. These include Kirpens Island (2), Crotched Pond Island (12), Moose Island (20), John Mack Bay (28), and a small nameless island off Long Island (32). Families and groups will often book neighboring sites at some of the multisite islands, including Doherty Island (7 and 8), Green Island (9 and 10), Camp Island (15–18), and Long Island (35–40), the largest of the bunch. Surprisingly, the most coveted site is not even on an island. Site 11, found near Watch Point, sits at the tip of a small peninsula, and promises campers their own beach and even a nearby waterfall.

Site 11 and the desirable island sites are often booked when they first become available—nine months in advance. But other lakeshore sites should not be overlooked.

:: Key Information

ADDRESS: NY 30, Sabael, NY 12864

OPERATED BY: New York State Department of Environmental Conservation

CONTACT: 518-648-5300; www.dec.ny .gov/outdoor/24471.html

OPEN: Mid-May–early October

SITES: 55

SITE AMENITIES: Picnic table and fire ring

ASSIGNMENT: Choose from available sites or reservations

REGISTRATION: On arrival or by reservation

FACILITIES: Pit toilets

PARKING: Central lot, near registration booth and boat launch

FEE: $20/night

ELEVATION: 1,670'

RESTRICTIONS:

■ **Pets:** Dogs on leash with proof of currently valid rabies vaccination

■ **Fires:** In fire rings only

■ **Alcohol:** At site

■ **Vehicles:** None permitted; sites are accessible only by boat.

■ **Other:** Quiet hours 10 p.m.–7 a.m.; carry out all trash

■ **Reservations:** 2-night stay required

They are ideal for those of us who don't mark up calendars, and they tend to be more densely wooded, giving the impression of having the wilderness all to yourself. If you are looking for the quietest sites, consider 42–51, at the southernmost end of the lake. Many boats will pass by 52–55, but these four convenient sites are the closest to the registration booth and boat launch, a selling point for less-seasoned paddlers.

Canoes and kayaks are certainly popular, but motorboats can make distant points on the lake more accessible, and considering this is a carry-in/carry-out facility, they make ferrying supplies easier. There are no restrictions on the types of boats allowed, but there are also no docks at the sites. The lake is not marked and there are many submerged rocks. Losing a propeller is no way to start a camping trip. And be sure to arrive early. The steep launch is the only public one on the lake, so it gets plenty of day use and the parking lot can overflow.

Waterskiing is best enjoyed at the north end of the lake, but great fishing

spots are everywhere. Trout, bass, and landlocked salmon attract many anglers. Some of the lakeshore is designated for picnicking, and both campers and day-use visitors take boats to trails that start right along the water's edge. On the eastern side of the lake are three 1-mile trails leading to Baldface Mountain, Crotched Pond, and John Mack Pond. Just north of the campground entrance on Route 30 is a trail leading more than 4 miles to Snowy Mountain. Across the highway is the Watch Hill Trail, which climbs to great views of the lake on Watch Hill.

On their way in or out of Indian Lake Islands, many campers take advantage of the showers and lifeguarded beach at Lewey Lake (no extra cost for those carrying their camping receipt). Others arriving too late to make their way to an Indian Lake site in the dark sometimes choose to use Lewey Lake as a stopover for the night. Just be warned that on summer weekends Lewey can fill to capacity, and you may have no choice but to find other accommodations.

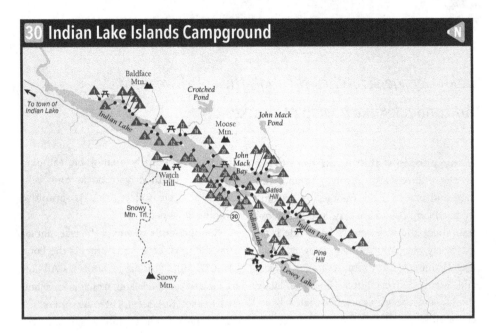

30 Indian Lake Islands Campground

Before the Indian Lake Islands Campground officially opened in 1960, Indian Lake had long been home to informal campsites. With no official oversight, heavy tree cutting, accumulation of trash, and forest fires left scars on the shorelines. These days, under the watchful eye of the DEC, these problems are no longer common. Though it may seem inconvenient to haul your own trash, think of how much you appreciate pitching a tent at a clean, rustic site after a day of boating.

:: Getting There

From I-87 (Adirondack Northway), take Exit 23, Warrensburg. Follow US 9 North 4 miles to NY 28, then follow NY 28 West 33 miles. In Indian Lake Village, take NY 30 South 12 miles. The campground entrance is on the left.

GPS COORDINATES   N43° 39.067'   W74° 23.383'

31

Lake George Islands

Lake George stretches through the southwestern Adirondacks like a wisp of smoke.

Many people's childhood memories of the Adirondacks revolve around the long and narrow Lake George. Its proximity to Albany, New York City, and even Boston (about 200 miles away) has made it an extremely popular summer getaway. Children's summer camps, rental cottages, lodges, and many budget motels line the lake's shores, and the water itself delights boaters of all stripes. Thirty-two miles long and 3 miles wide at its widest point, Lake George stretches through the southwestern Adirondacks like a wisp of smoke. And islands, some acres-large and others little more than rocks sprouting a few trees, pop up across the water. You could camp along the shores at Roger's Rock or Hearthstone Point, but with almost 400 prime campsites to choose from on the lake's roughly 150 islands, why bother?

Lake George Islands is actually divided into three campgrounds (or groups) with three separate headquarters: the Long Island Group (LI); Glen Island Group (GI); and the Narrow Island Group (NI). But it is hard to choose one group over another, and each

site offers an equally memorable camping experience. With private docks and well-maintained pit toilets, this is primitive camping at its best.

On the southern end of the lake, not far from the town of Lake George, is the Long Island Group, featuring 90 campsites. All sites are located on one island, which is large and shaped like a turkey leg. There are some small islands nearby for exploring and picnicking, including Diamond and Specker Heck, which have day-use areas—but your tent will have to stay put on Long Island. This does not mean you will feel cramped and overrun with neighbors. The campground staff has done a great job throughout the lake keeping all the islands well wooded and the sites well spaced. You will see other campers during your visit to Long Island, but this will not distract from the beauty of the surroundings.

Farther north, in The Narrows of the lake, is the Glen Island Group. With its central location and 170 sites, it tends to be quite busy. Single-site islands (Bass, Gourd, Hermit, Little Gourd, Perch, Pine, Refuge, and Sunny) are unquestionably prime property. There are also larger islands that each house two to five sites, perfect for groups. The largest islands, such as Big Burnt with its 28 sites and Turkey with its 33, tend to be easier to book on short notice. The group also features the lake's only cruiser sites. Located along the eastern shore at Red Rock Bay and on Log Bay Island, these 42 sites feature

:: Ratings

BEAUTY: ★ ★ ★ ★ ★
PRIVACY: ★ ★ ★ ★
QUIET: ★ ★ ★ ★
CLEANLINESS: ★ ★ ★ ★
SECURITY: ★ ★ ★ ★ ★
SPACIOUSNESS: ★ ★ ★ ★ ★

:: Key Information

ADDRESS: 18 Boathouse Ln., Bolton Landing, NY 12814

OPERATED BY: New York State Department of Environmental Conservation

CONTACT: GI sites, 518-644-9696; LI sites, 518-656-9426; NI sites, 518-499-1288; www.dec.ny.gov/outdoor/24474.html

OPEN: Mid-May–early October

SITES: Glen Island, 212; Long Island, 90; Narrow Island, 85

SITE AMENITIES: Picnic table, fire ring, dock, and toilet facility; 42 sites for large boats with sleeping quarters also have charcoal burners and pit toilets.

ASSIGNMENT: Choose from available sites or reservations

REGISTRATION: On-site, by reservation

FACILITIES: Pit toilets

PARKING: At private marinas; fee usually charged

FEE: $28/night

ELEVATION: 320'

RESTRICTIONS:
- **Pets:** No dogs
- **Fires:** In fire rings only
- **Alcohol:** At site
- **Vehicles:** None permitted; sites are accessible only by boat.
- **Other:** Quiet hours 10 p.m.–7 a.m.; carry out all trash
- **Reservations:** GI and NI, 3-night stay required (LI, 1-night stay allowed)

larger docks, designed for boats with sleeping quarters. Think of this as the RV section of the lake. Tent campers need not bother booking any of these—this area is mainly for people who want to sleep in the cabins of their boats.

The 85 sites of the Narrow Island Group are actually located north of The Narrows, which may be a little confusing. Just remember that this group (also known as the Mother Bunch), stretches throughout the entire north half of the lake from just south of Huletts Landing almost the entire way to Ticonderoga. The islands are smaller in this neck of the water, and although single-site islands (Coopers, Horicon, Little Burgess, Mallory, Phenita, and Steere) should not be passed up, only St. Sacrament, with 19 sites, could even be close to crowded.

Describing each individual site on Lake George would require an entire book. ReserveAmerica has done some of the work for us and provides distinct descriptions of

each campsite, including details about water depth, foliage, and views. Pay careful attention to these options if you require a tent platform or have certain requirements for your boat. And a handful of sites are non-reservable—good for last-minute planners.

Before choosing a site, you should assess what your boat can handle. Although kayaks and canoes are common on Lake George, motorboats are the dominant form of transport. When the weather gets dicey, the wind often kicks up whitecaps on the lake, and paddlers may find themselves in danger. Campground staff told us tales of people with kayaks and canoes being stranded at their sites because of bad weather.

All three campground headquarters are located on islands (Glen, Long, and Narrow): you may have to travel a few miles over open water to check in, and then another few miles to get to your site. Be sure to leave yourself plenty of time—you don't want to rush, especially late in the evening

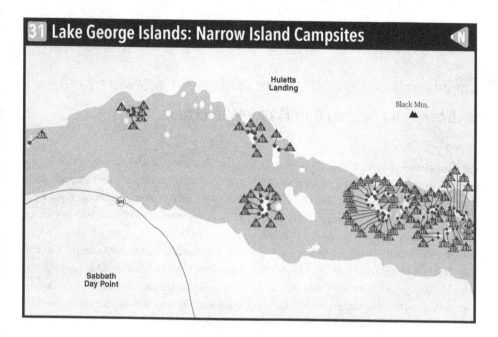

31 Lake George Islands: Narrow Island Campsites

or if you are not confident in your boating abilities. No official boat launches access any of the campgrounds. The best option is to find a local marina and pay a small fee to park and launch. If you are renting a boat, this makes things quite convenient. But if you are bringing your own, it is a bit of an annoyance. Make sure to pick up a map and/or hydrographic chart at the marina, because the lake does hold many submerged rocks. For information on marinas, go to **visitlakegeorge.com,** or contact the campground offices or the Warren County Tourism Department at 518-761-6366.

:: Getting There

Drive to Lake George from I-87 (Adirondack Northway) using Exits 21–25 and 28, then NY 9, NY 9N, NY 8, or NY 74. Contact a local marina for specific driving directions to your chosen boat launch (see phone number and website above), and steer your vessel toward the island headquarters using the GPS coordinates below.

GPS COORDINATES (LONG ISLAND HEADQUARTERS)
N43° 29.067'   W73° 39.217'

GPS COORDINATES (GLEN ISLAND HEADQUARTERS)
N43° 34.383'   W73° 36.050'

GPS COORDINATES (NARROW ISLAND HEADQUARTERS)
N43° 38.750'   W73° 30.417'

32

Lake Harris

Lake Harris is one of the more convenient gateways to the southern end of the High Peaks Wilderness.

As you drive to Lake Harris Campground on the curvy mountain road known as NY Route 28, look for signs depicting the silhouette of a man with glasses and a moustache. That's Theodore Roosevelt, all right. While camping on Mount Marcy on September 14, 1901, Teddy received word that President William McKinley had been shot and was not expected to recover. His party quickly hiked 10 miles down to Long Lake and Roosevelt continued west in a frantic nighttime stagecoach ride to the nearest train station. Arriving in North Creek, he discovered that McKinley had died and that he was now president.

In commemoration of this legendary journey, Route 28 is known today as the Roosevelt–Marcy Trail. Roosevelt was, of course, a legendary outdoorsman and went on to become instrumental in the creation of the national park system. The Adirondacks didn't need his help, though: they were already preserved, thanks to a state law passed in 1885. The Adirondack Park continues to be larger than any national park in the continental United States.

:: Ratings

BEAUTY: ★ ★ ★ ★
PRIVACY: ★ ★ ★
QUIET: ★ ★ ★ ★
CLEANLINESS: ★ ★ ★
SECURITY: ★ ★
SPACIOUSNESS: ★ ★ ★ ★

Like many of the campgrounds in the region, Lake Harris offers waterfront sites, but in a much higher percentage than what is typically available. Almost two-thirds are along the water—57 out of 89—and all are well shaded by tall hardwoods. The first sites along the dirt road (1–5) are among the finest—large, private, and well spaced. More-congested spaces follow, but they are still adequately distributed, with sites 52 and 69 providing the most solitude. Sites 60, 76–79, 81, 83, and 90 are the least desirable, but the point is almost moot. Lake Harris is not an especially popular campground, and except for holidays it is rarely busy. Whether you have a reservation or not, you should have plenty of sites from which to choose.

Fed by the northern part of the Hudson River, Lake Harris has 275 surface acres. While swimming is not allowed at the campground, campers do certainly take advantage of the water. There is a small boat ramp just past the registration booth and larger public ramps elsewhere on the lake. Motorboats are allowed, but only canoes and kayaks are available to rent. Bass, yellow perch, and northern pike will keep anglers casting their lines. Wildlife abounds in the surrounding woods, and although sightings of moose are extremely rare, bears are seen regularly. Please follow campground precautions concerning food storage and trash disposal.

Lake Harris is one of the more convenient gateways to the southern end of the

:: Key Information

ADDRESS: NY 28, North Newcomb, NY 12852

OPERATED BY: New York State Department of Environmental Conservation

CONTACT: 518-582-2503; www.dec.ny .gov/outdoor/24469.html

OPEN: Mid-May–early September

SITES: 89

SITE AMENITIES: Picnic table and fire ring

ASSIGNMENT: Choose from available sites

REGISTRATION: On arrival or by reservation

FACILITIES: Water, flush toilets, showers

PARKING: At site, maximum 2 vehicles

FEE: $18/night

ELEVATION: 1,611'

RESTRICTIONS:

■ **Pets:** Dogs on leash with proof of currently valid rabies vaccination

■ **Fires:** In fire rings only

■ **Alcohol:** At site

■ **Vehicles:** Up to 40'

■ **Other:** Quiet hours 10 p.m.–7 a.m.; no swimming

■ **Reservations:** 1-night stay allowed

High Peaks Wilderness, with major trailheads located in the ghost town of Tahawus, about a 25-minute drive to the north. Some of the more celebrated hikes, such as Mount Marcy and Mount Algonquin, are closer to Lake Placid. Yet many folks will find it preferable to stay at Lake Harris and log a little time in the car in order to avoid the zoo that is Lake Placid in the summer. Closer to the campground, a 2-mile hike up Goodnow Mountain, capped by a fire tower, is a nice option for families who are ready for the 1,000-foot rise. The steepest part of the trail is in the beginning, and benches along the way provide convenient places to rest. The nearby climb to Vanderwacker Mountain also leads to a fire tower, and at 5 miles round-trip, it is a little more challenging than Goodnow, but nothing more than a moderate day hike.

In addition to a monument commemorating Roosevelt's historic ride, a number of attractions in the vicinity of Lake Harris allow you to learn more about the Adirondacks' 6 million acres. Newcomb houses one of the two Adirondack Park Interpretive Centers (the other is in Paul Smiths), where indoor exhibits are complemented by miles of surfaced nature trails. The Camp Santanoni Historic Area can be reached by foot, bike, or car. A trail beginning at the edge of the campground leads 1.5 miles to the preserve and 6.5 miles to Camp Santanoni's main lodge, or "great camp," which provides a fascinating perspective into the past, when the Adirondacks were being discovered as a playground for the rich who wanted the amenities of large homes but the feeling of true wilderness. During the summer, a number of the buildings are open to visitors, while the preserve itself is open year-round. Finally, 25 miles to the west in Blue Mountain Lake, you can visit the Adirondack Museum, with exhibits depicting the rough-and-tumble history and culture of the mountains.

With the High Peaks close at hand and so many opportunities to learn about the natural and human history of the Adirondacks, Lake Harris is an ideal campground for the adventurous. You may not stick around your site for long, but when you do, you'll appreciate the serenity that attracted Roosevelt and so many others over the years.

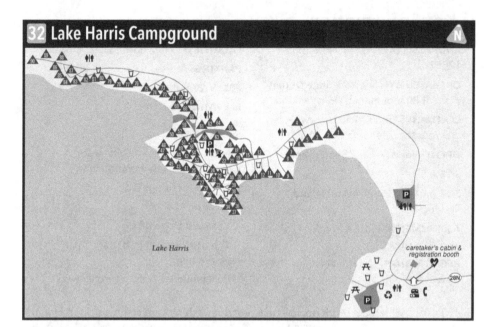

:: Getting There

From I-87 (Adirondack Northway), take Exit 23 to NY 9 South and follow it 4.5 miles to NY 28. Then drive 16 miles northwest to North Creek and take NY 28N 24.5 miles to Newcomb. The campground entrance is on the right.

GPS COORDINATES N43° 58.517' W74° 07.467'

33

Lincoln Pond

Campers can exit the major highway and be setting up tents within 30 minutes.

Lincoln Pond and its small campground are located just east of the Adirondack Northway (I-87). Surrounded by privately owned land, the pond and campground offer few trails for hikers (you will have to travel west into the Giant Mountain Wilderness to summit a few peaks). What they do offer, however, are some of the most beautiful campsites in the state.

A causeway separates Lincoln Pond into Upper and Lower Ponds, connecting the land at the water's narrowest point. From here, some of the campsites are visible, while "camps," the Adirondack term for summer homes or cottages, can be seen across the water. The terminology dates back to the early 1800s, when many Americans first discovered the joys of the Adirondacks, which were becoming an increasingly accessible wilderness. Even the grandest compounds are still called camps, but thankfully most of the camps on Lincoln Pond are just modest family homes. The famed "great camps," the grandest of these compounds, are farther to the west. So don't be confused if a local

:: Ratings

BEAUTY: ★ ★ ★
PRIVACY: ★ ★ ★
QUIET: ★ ★ ★
CLEANLINESS: ★ ★ ★ ★
SECURITY: ★ ★ ★ ★
SPACIOUSNESS: ★ ★ ★

tells you he or she is "going to camp" for the weekend. They may have no intention of pitching a tent or firing up an RV.

A kayak, canoe, or small motorboat will undoubtedly enhance a visit to Lincoln Pond. Its gentle waters are great for an afternoon paddle or fishing for smallmouth bass, tiger muskie, and bullhead. There is no need to worry if you do not own a boat. The campground rents canoes and rowboats for a reasonable fee. You should worry about reservations, though. For although the main campground is full of fine waterfront sites, it is the primitive and island (also known as interior) sites that make it worth a visit, and eager campers reserve them months in advance.

With the exception of site 35R, each of these other 10 sites borders the water. The closest of these to the main campground are 26R–28R, accessible by car from Lincoln Pond Road. Of the first three, 28R is the most private. Each has a picnic table, fire ring, and pit toilets, but no running water. Campers have to return to the main area for water or a shower. This is a mild hassle and a short drive, but well worth it for the isolation. Three more sites (29R–31R) are located on a small wooded island on Upper Pond, and boaters book these far in advance. Less than 2 miles down Lincoln Pond Road, turn right onto Kingdom Dam Road and drive for about 1 mile to reach sites 32R–35R. These are all excellent places to pitch a tent, but if

:: Key Information

ADDRESS: 4363 Lincoln Pond Rd., Elizabethtown, NY 12932

OPERATED BY: New York State Department of Environmental Conservation

CONTACT: 518-942-5292; www.dec.ny .gov/outdoor/24477.html

OPEN: Mid-May-early September

SITES: 35 (including 7 primitive drive-in sites and 3 boat-in sites)

SITE AMENITIES: Picnic table and fire ring

ASSIGNMENT: Choose from available sites or reservations

REGISTRATION: On arrival or by reservation

FACILITIES: Water, pit and flush toilets, showers, beach, picnic area, boat launch

PARKING: At site, maximum 2 vehicles or designated lot for walk-in and boat-in sites

FEE: $18/night

ELEVATION: 1,060'

RESTRICTIONS:

■ Pets: Dogs on leash with proof of currently valid rabies vaccination

■ Fires: In fire rings only

■ Alcohol: At site

■ Vehicles: Up to 30'

■ Other: Quiet hours 10 p.m.–7 a.m.

■ Reservations: 1-night stay allowed

we had to choose one site, it would be 34R. Perched on soft earth above the northern end of Lincoln Pond, it offers wonderful views, easy access to the water, and a spacious spot to hang a hammock, stow a boat, and enjoy a quiet day.

Back at Lincoln Pond's main camping area, you can take advantage of the day-use beach, picnic area, and car-top boat launch. Two nearby DEC campgrounds, Sharp Bridge and Crown Point, do not offer swimming, so some of their campers are likely to join locals at the beach here on hot days. The sand slopes down to the water, offering some very attractive spots to hunker down in a lawn chair and enjoy the surroundings.

The 25 sites in the main campground are rather open, with the waterfront sites being the least private (only a few birches and pines separate campers from their neighbors). But considering you can basically stick your feet out of your tent and dip them right into the water, try to reserve ahead (recommended for all sites on weekends and holidays) for 1,

2, 4, 6, 7, 9, 10, 12, 13, or 15. The last site along the water, 15, is spacious but very close to the causeway. Number 12 is on an embankment, so it is flat. The sites not directly on the water are also flat, but perched upon a slope, providing water views. The most private sites are 21 and 22. Site 23 is sunny and removed from the others, but is surrounded by an open field with an access road passing through, so it doesn't offer as much privacy as one might expect from the map.

Nearby Elizabethtown is a good place to pick up supplies and is home to the Adirondack History Center, an excellent small museum. Here you'll find displays on recreation in the region and a number of restored vehicles, ranging from a brightly painted stagecoach to a hand-pump fire truck to a 1932 Olympics bobsled. One of its most popular attractions is the nearly 60-foot-high restored fire observation tower that you can climb for views of the town and the surrounding forest.

Bordered by I-87 to the west and Lake Champlain to the east, this section of the

Adirondacks is more accessible than most. Campers can exit the interstate and be setting up tents within 30 minutes. And even with private "camps" on the shores of the lake, the sense of one's own space is still strong. Forest Preserve regulations limit development, and there are unlikely to be any major hotels constructed on the lake anytime soon. The privacy and accessibility of Lincoln Pond's interior sites make them even more desirable for tent campers. If you can plan ahead, it's worth the wait to get one of these well-planned spaces, whether for a couple's weekend getaway or a two-week family vacation.

:: Getting There

From I-87 (Adirondack Northway), take Exit 31, Elizabethtown, and follow NY 9N west 4 miles. Turn left on CR 7 (Lincoln Pond Road) and go 6 miles to the campground entrance on the right.

GPS COORDINATES   N44° 08.400'   W73° 34.683'

34

Little Sand Point

It is likely that campers will have the concrete boat ramp and sandy beach all to themselves.

Almost 5 miles long and 1 mile wide, Piseco Lake in Hamilton County is one of many bodies of water created when the last ice age retreated. Today, summer homes and year-round retreats dot its shores. Luckily for tent campers, there are also three campgrounds on the lake's western edge. Our favorite of the three is Little Sand Point.

Poplar Point, near the northwestern corner of Piseco, is the smallest and oldest of the three, and features pit toilets and 21 sites along marshy water. It was built in 1927 and became so popular that the Department of Conservation quickly built Point Comfort, an area on the southwestern corner of the lake with pit toilets and 76 sites crowded together in what looks like a large picnic area. The aptly named Little Sand Point, built in 1953 and located between the other two, has the smallest beach and some relatively small sites, but it has the prettiest views, the most privacy, and the newest facilities (flush toilets, if that matters to you). We recommend you choose Little Sand for a stay on Piseco. All three campgrounds offer boat launches

and beaches, but Little Sand is the farthest from town, and its facilities are rarely visited by day-trippers, so campers likely will have the concrete boat ramp and sandy beach all to themselves.

Across from the entrance to the campground is the recycling center and dump station, wisely separated from the main area by County Route 8. The registration booth sits just past the gate, and a single road follows the shoreline past all 78 sites, with a circle at the far end to turn around. Slightly more than half of the spaces border the water, but trees block some of the views. These mixed hardwoods and conifers contribute a great deal of shade and a strong sense of privacy, and even if the sites seem small at first in comparison to other campgrounds in the Adirondacks, you will quickly find them to be more than adequate for a tent or two.

The first couple of sites are situated a little too close to the beach and boat ramp for comfort. Skip those. Most any of the other lakeside sites will do, and even though they are located on a gentle slope, there are plenty of flat patches to pitch a tent. If you have your choice, try sites 50–65, the best for tents at Little Sand. Large rocks block the entrances to these sites, preventing cars from entering. Campers park along the road and walk the 10 yards or so to pitch a tent. Vehicles are still easily accessible, but anyone camping in this section can be guaranteed a bit more privacy.

:: Ratings

BEAUTY: ★ ★ ★
PRIVACY: ★ ★ ★ ★
QUIET: ★ ★ ★ ★ ★
CLEANLINESS: ★ ★ ★ ★
SECURITY: ★ ★
SPACIOUSNESS: ★ ★ ★

:: Key Information

ADDRESS: Old Piseco Road, Piseco, NY 12139

OPERATED BY: New York State Department of Environmental Conservation

CONTACT: 518-548-7585; www.dec.ny .gov/outdoor/24479.html

OPEN: Mid-May–early September

SITES: 78

SITE AMENITIES: Picnic table and fire ring

ASSIGNMENT: Choose from available sites or reservations

REGISTRATION: On arrival or by reservation

FACILITIES: Water, flush toilets, showers, pay phone

PARKING: At site, maximum 2 vehicles

FEE: $20/night

ELEVATION: 1,668'

RESTRICTIONS:

■ **Pets:** Dogs on leash with proof of currently valid rabies vaccination

■ **Fires:** In fire rings only

■ **Alcohol:** At site

■ **Vehicles:** Up to 30'

■ **Other:** Quiet hours 10 p.m.–7 a.m.

■ **Reservations:** 2-night stay required

The nearby village of Piseco offers few supplies. Drive a little farther to Speculator, where the kitschy sign reading WELCOME TO SPECULATOR—ALL SEASON VACATIONLAND greets you. It is one of the area's larger villages, but considering that the population hovers around 350, that's not saying a lot. Still, there are spots for lunch and dinner, and a handful of inns and motels. It is a community that depends on visitors.

Closer to the campground, along County Route 8, a short trail affords excellent views of Piseco Lake. It meanders about 0.8 mile up to Panther Mountain's 700-foot-high Echo Cliffs. The 5-mile T Lake Trail, climbing nearly 1,000 feet from Poplar Point Campground, might be a better choice if you crave longer distances. And, if that's not enough for you, hop on a section of the 133-mile Northville–Placid Trail at the northern tip of the lake. You'll be catching it at about the 30-mile point, so there is plenty more ground to cover.

Many campers (and others) take advantage of the lake and fish for dinner (or just for fun). Lake and brook trout, common and round whitefish, brown bullhead, chain pickerel, yellow perch, smallmouth bass, yellow perch, and pumpkinseed are all found in Piseco Lake. The lake itself can accommodate all sorts of boats. Motorboats, sailboats, canoes, and kayaks skim along the water on clear summer days. If campers get bored with the beach at Little Sand Point, they can enjoy the sometimes-quieter Poplar Point Beach or the busier Point Comfort Beach. But always check in advance to see if any lifeguards are on duty—they can be hard to come by in this neck of the woods.

Private homes share the western edge of the lake with the campground. You may spy summer visitors looking out over the blue water and green forests from their comfortable, weathered Adirondack chairs. It is easy to see why this characteristic type of outdoor furniture, with its sloping back and wide armrests, is named after the region: an Adirondack chair, like the mountains themselves, evokes a slow pace and simple, natural pleasures. Back at Sandy Point, you may have to make do with a well-worn picnic-table bench. It's a small sacrifice for a quiet night in this pleasant little getaway on the water.

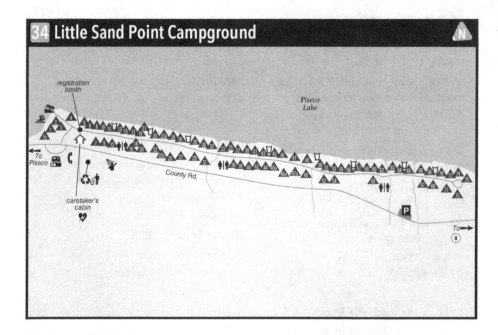

:: Getting There

From I-90 (New York State Thruway), take Exit 27, Amsterdam, to NY 30 North and follow it 50 miles. In Speculator, turn left on NY 8 West. After 11 miles, turn right on Old Piseco Road and follow it 5 miles. The campground entrance is on the left.

GPS COORDINATES   N43° 25.050'   W74° 33.100'

35

Luzerne

Two corrals, a barn, and miles of horse trails round out the benefits for equestrians.

Straddling the "blue line" marking the border of the Adirondack Park, the town of Lake Luzerne is known as the "Gateway to the Adirondacks," and Luzerne campground is just inside this boundary. Like much of the area, the surrounding forest was once owned by a lumber company and heavily logged in the 1940s and '50s. When the state purchased the land in the 1960s, horse trails were already established on the property. Now the trees are thick again, and this pleasant campground has the unique features of horse camping and two separate swimming areas—one reserved for campers only.

After entering Luzerne, turn left and pass the boat launch to reach the campsites. The first section (sites 1–15) is set in dense, shady forest with beds of pine needles that beckon you to unfurl your tent. Removed from the other loops, this section promises the most quiet. Sites 7–11, down a short hill on a small, secluded spur, are the ones to choose here. Skip sites 4 and 12–15, which are a little too close to the road. Beyond the first section, the camp road curves, crossing

a stream and the "Field of Dreams," a grassy clearing perfect for a lazy picnic. The next section of sites (16–37) is larger and also isolated, but draws bigger crowds. Ferns are thick in this section, and site 22, carved a little deeper than the others into the forest, was our favorite here.

Another short drive down the road leads to the next section, by far the largest with more than half the sites in the campground. Sites 38–123 are arranged in a group of intersecting loops, and many centrally located spaces have their own entrances but neighbors on the other three sides. On the campground map, sites 81, 82, 113, 114, 116, and 118 appear to be close to the water's edge and the beach, so they tend to book up quickly. But they are atop a steep hill. Don't expect to fall asleep to the sound of lapping water here. Number 94 is one of the more private spots; 119, 120, and 120A are set off on a spur near a ravine.

From the small parking lot near site number 113, it's just a 50-yard walk down to the campers' beach. This small patch of sand lies across the lake from the day-use bathing area. Both have lifeguards on duty during summer days. The campers' beach is the smaller of the two, but is quieter and has its own rowboats and canoes for rent. It is nice to see that your camping pass can get you more than just a patch of dirt and a fire pit. Even if you're not a sun worshiper, the beach is still a relaxing spot to take in the views of the wooded slopes surrounding the water.

:: Ratings

BEAUTY: ★ ★ ★
PRIVACY: ★ ★ ★
QUIET: ★ ★ ★ ★
CLEANLINESS: ★ ★ ★
SECURITY: ★ ★ ★
SPACIOUSNESS: ★ ★ ★

:: Key Information

ADDRESS: 892 Lake Ave. (NY 9N), Lake Luzerne, NY 12846

OPERATED BY: New York State Department of Environmental Conservation

CONTACT: 518-696-2031; www.dec.ny .gov/outdoor/24480.html

OPEN: Mid-May–early September

SITES: 174

SITE AMENITIES: Picnic table and fire ring

ASSIGNMENT: Choose from available sites or reservations

REGISTRATION: On arrival or by reservation

FACILITIES: Water, flush toilets, hot showers

PARKING: At site, maximum 2 vehicles

FEE: $22/night

ELEVATION: 620'

RESTRICTIONS:

■ **Pets:** Dogs on leash with proof of currently valid rabies vaccination; horses permitted with proof of a currently valid negative Coggins test for equine infectious anemia

■ **Fires:** In fire rings only

■ **Alcohol:** At site

■ **Vehicles:** Up to 30' in main section, up to 40' in horse section

■ **Other:** Quiet hours 10 p.m.–7 a.m.

■ **Reservations:** 2-night stay required

Leaving the main group of sites, you pass the campground's shower building. Comfort stations and water spigots are well spaced throughout the campground, but this is the only place for a shower, and thankfully it features a small parking lot. Turn right after the showers and onto the main road, and you will come to the next group of sites (124–150). Though these are nicely removed from the largest section, power lines crisscross overhead and seem incongruous to the wooded surroundings. It would be quite pleasant here if it weren't for the constant reminder of civilization.

The final section is made up of the equestrian sites (H1–H22). Although this area is essentially an open field surrounded by pines, campers with horses will appreciate not having to book extra sites. Two corrals, a barn, and miles of horse trails round out the benefits for equestrians. There are only 5 miles of equine trails within the surrounding public land, but more than 60 miles are accessible on adjacent private property—detailed on a posted map. On holiday weekends, you must have a horse to stay in this area.

The lake itself is known as Fourth Lake, a testament to the sheer number of lakes in the Adirondacks—they ran out of names and had to settle for numbers! Second and Third Lakes are to the south, and Lake Luzerne is actually a separate and much larger body of water found in town. Fourth Lake is only partially bordered by the campground but is still a quiet bit of water where no motorboats are allowed. The day-use area is popular for swimming, picnicking, and fishing. Canoes and rowboats are also available for rent at the beach. The park staff runs a nature recreation program—check the posted *Wilderness Times,* a summary of daily events written by the camp staff in the summer.

Even if you don't own a horse, you can still have a cowboy experience nearby. Just follow the Dude Ranch Trail signs north on 9N, and in minutes you'll be at the Painted Pony Rodeo. Barbecue dinners and rodeo

35 Luzerne Campground

shows rope in everyone from cowboys to greenhorns. For a shopping and dining blitz, continue on to Lake George and its honky-tonk attractions. There are campgrounds on the shores of Lake George, but they are even larger than Luzerne's, and tent campers should avoid them in summer (the Lake George Islands campgrounds [see page 108] are another story). Luzerne is much quieter and almost as close to the action. If you avoid the largest section of sites, it's hard even to believe that you are camping in such a big campground. The facilities are well worn but clean, a testament to the many people who have enjoyed the campground over the years.

:: Getting There

From I-87 (Adirondack Northway), take Exit 21 to NY 9N South, and follow it 7 miles to the campground entrance, on the left.

GPS COORDINATES   N43° 21.617'   W73° 49.000'

36

Meacham Lake

What makes Meacham Lake stand out is the presence of a separate, undeveloped area filled with tent-only camping, including two dozen walk-in sites.

In the far northwest corner of the Adirondacks sits Meacham Lake, one of the most remote campgrounds in the state. In many ways, it is similar to other campgrounds in the mountains, with its calm, clear waters dotted with coveted campsites, and its mix of firs and hardwoods shading the tents, trailers, and RVs that overrun it every summer weekend. What makes Meacham Lake stand out is the presence of a separate, undeveloped area filled with tent-only camping, including two dozen walk-in sites. Known as Meacham Lake West (to be honest, the name reminds us of a new housing development), this isolated mini-campground is perfect for those who want to get away from it all but still have their cars only a short walk away.

The main camping area at Meacham is large and fairly standard, but we do not want to downplay its appeal. It includes a day-use area with a picnic shelter, sandy beach, playground, and canoes and rowboats for rent. The closest major towns are Malone and Saranac Lakes (20 miles to the north and south, respectively), so campers rarely have to contend with crowds of day-use visitors. One of the unique features of the campground is the large amphitheater found east of the beach, on the southern side of the shower-house parking lot. With seating for up to 100 people, it serves as a venue for educational and recreational activities (including movies and even the occasional karaoke session). For daily events in the summer, look for the posted *Wilderness Times* newsletter or talk to the camp staff.

If privacy is the most important aspect of a campsite for you, seek out sites 25–33, 72, or 73, which are spacious and set deeper into the woods than most. Avoid sites 1–5, 42–44, 53–55, and 84–91. They are crowded, and not as shady as one might like. The waterfront sites (153–174) are obviously the most popular, and visitors will appreciate that there is no private development on the lake to spoil the views. Especially for waterfront sites, reservations on weekends and holidays are essential, but walk-in campers should not have problems during the week if they are happy with a standard site.

According to the camp staff, Meacham Lake West is the last area that fills up by advance request. Removed from the main campground and day-use area, it is about a mile past the boat ramp via a paved road (though that doesn't mean it isn't free of the

:: Ratings

BEAUTY: ★ ★ ★ ★
PRIVACY: ★ ★ ★ ★
QUIET: ★ ★ ★ ★
CLEANLINESS: ★ ★ ★
SECURITY: ★ ★ ★ ★
SPACIOUSNESS: ★ ★ ★ ★

:: Key Information

ADDRESS: 119 State Campsite Rd., Duane, NY 12953

OPERATED BY: New York State Department of Environmental Conservation

CONTACT: 518-483-5116; www.dec.ny.gov/outdoor/24481.html

OPEN: Late June–early October

SITES: 224 (48 primitive, including 24 walk-in)

SITE AMENITIES: Picnic table and fire ring (walk-in sites also have tent platforms)

ASSIGNMENT: Choose from available sites or reservations

REGISTRATION: On arrival or by reservation

FACILITIES: Water (potable water not available at walk-in sites), pit and flush toilets, showers, pay phone

PARKING: At site or designated areas for walk-ins, maximum 2 vehicles

FEE: $20/night

ELEVATION: 1,573'

RESTRICTIONS:

■ **Pets:** Dogs on leash with proof of currently valid rabies vaccination

■ **Fires:** In fire rings only

■ **Alcohol:** At site

■ **Vehicles:** Up to 40'

■ **Other:** Quiet hours 10 p.m.–7 a.m.

■ **Reservations:** 1-night stay allowed

occasional pothole). When the road turns to dirt, you have to park your car and hoof it to access the best sites. If that's not enough to keep the trailers away, the fact that only one collection of pit toilets services the 50 sites will do the trick.

Sites 175–199 are all primitive walk-in sites, but the walk to each varies from about 30 to 300 yards. All sites are either on the water or open to excellent views—each has its own outhouse and tent platform. The facilities may be a little old, and the lakeshore sites are not completely private (other sites can often be seen through the trees), but they are a vast improvement over most accommodations a tent camper is likely to find. For those who would like to take advantage of the remoteness of Meacham Lake West, but would prefer the proximity of a few more amenities, sites 201–223 are spread out along a separate road and are closest to the toilets and a series of water spigots. Sites 179–181 sit atop a grassy hill and would be perfect for group camping.

A firewood and ice truck peddles the basics to campers once a day (more frequently in the summer). For other supplies, the closest store is a 6-mile drive north out of the campground along New York State Route 30. But a little time on the road is not such a bad thing around here. NY 30, a scenic byway known as the Adirondack Trail, is one of the nicest stretches of road in the state. Follow it almost 10 miles south to the village of Paul Smiths, home to Paul Smith's College, known for its programs in forestry, ecology, and hospitality. The village is also home to one of the two Adirondack Park Visitor Interpretive Centers (the other is in Newcomb), a great place to learn about the region through wildlife exhibits, scheduled events, and miles of surfaced trails designed for those not quite ready for backcountry hiking.

From Paul Smiths, hikers can summit St. Regis Mountain, a 2,874-foot peak that overlooks the St. Regis Canoe Area. Those who would rather not drive to a trailhead

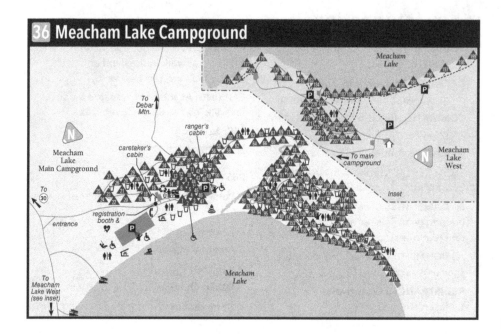

36 Meacham Lake Campground

can set off from the campground and climb Debar Mountain, a 7.4-mile round-trip that will take you up to 3,200 feet, the best vantage point in the Debar Mountain Wild Forest.

It may not be evident now, but the campground was built on the site of a well-known hotel that offered rooms to vacationers until 1921. The accommodations available at Meacham Lake these days are admittedly a bit more rustic, but the inviting sounds of nature and true feeling of wilderness should keep visitors coming back.

:: Getting There

From I-87 (Adirondack Northway), take Exit 30 to NY 73 North and follow it 28 miles. In Lake Placid, take NY 86 West for 22 miles, passing through the village of Saranac Lake. In Paul Smiths, turn right on NY 30 North and follow it 9.5 miles. The campground entrance is on the right.

GPS COORDINATES N44° 35.167' W74° 17.483'

37

Putnam Pond

Since the 1960s, it has provided quiet camping and tranquil waters for boaters wishing to escape the wakes of Lake George and Lake Champlain.

Fort Ticonderoga was once one of the most strategically important military sites in the New World. Built by the French in the 1750s and formerly called Fort Carillon, it's located at the point where Lake Champlain meets Lake George. It was known as the "key to the continent" and changed hands for its first 20 years between the French, the British, and the Americans. In 1820, it was privately purchased, and preservation of the site began. The fort, and the town that bears its name, still remain—but now the region, with its shimmering bodies of water, is more notable as a summer getaway, and the number of nearby campgrounds speaks to that fact. Paradox Lake, Crown Point, and Rogers Rock all provide camping within minutes of Ticonderoga. But Putnam Pond, just 6 miles down the road, features the finest accommodations for the tent camper.

Putnam Pond, known locally as Putts Pond, was originally named after General Israel Putnam, who gained notoriety as a

captain who fought in the region during the French and Indian War and later commanded forces at Bunker Hill. Since the campground's construction in the early 1960s, it has provided quiet camping and tranquil waters for boaters wishing to escape the wakes of Lake George and Lake Champlain. Unlike many campgrounds in the Adirondacks, it does not offer waterfront sites in its main campground. However, it does have a handful of boat-in and walk-in sites along its shores, and campers snatch these up quickly.

Putnam Creek, which flows from a dam on the east side of the pond and eventually runs into Lake Champlain, welcomes visitors as they drive over a bridge just past the entrance. The first sites, 1–16, are perfectly adequate but are a bit too close to the road for our tastes. Sites 17–34, on the north end of the campground, sold us on Putnam. We particularly liked site 28, which is shaded by large trees and set back along a slope, far from the road. Views of the pond are not as common as one might hope, but that enhances the feeling that you are in dense forest. For a glimpse of the water, choose site 46 or 47. Groups and large RVs are often directed to a grassy circle of sites (58–61) on the south side of the park, well removed from everyone else. And three "management" sites are maintained and often used

:: Ratings

BEAUTY: ★ ★ ★ ★
PRIVACY: ★ ★ ★ ★ ★
QUIET: ★ ★ ★
CLEANLINESS: ★ ★ ★ ★
SECURITY: ★ ★ ★ ★
SPACIOUSNESS: ★ ★ ★

:: Key Information

ADDRESS: 763 Putts Pond Rd., Ticonderoga, NY 12883

OPERATED BY: New York State Department of Environmental Conservation

CONTACT: 518-585-7280; www.dec.ny .gov/outdoor/24492.html

OPEN: Mid-May–early October

SITES: 72 (9 interior sites accessible only by boat)

SITE AMENITIES: Picnic table and fire ring

ASSIGNMENT: Choose from available sites or reservations

REGISTRATION: On arrival or by reservation

FACILITIES: Water (potable water not available at interior sites), pit and flush toilets, showers

PARKING: At site, maximum 2 vehicles or central lot for interior sites

FEE: $18/night

ELEVATION: 1,276'

RESTRICTIONS:

■ **Pets:** Dogs on leash with proof of currently valid rabies vaccination

■ **Fires:** In fire rings only

■ **Alcohol:** At site

■ **Vehicles:** Up to 30'

■ **Other:** Quiet hours 10 p.m.–7 a.m.

■ **Reservations:** 1-night stay allowed

for overflow. During the week, walk-ups should not have trouble finding vacancies, but weekends and holidays fill up quickly.

When we asked a staff member which sites are the most popular, she showed us her reservation sheet. The sites most frequently marked as booked happened to be the least accessible of the bunch, at least for the unfortunate folks without a boat or a sturdy pair of boots. The campground manages nine interior pond sites, including one on a small island (R-5). It is possible but difficult to hike in to sites R-8 and R-9 on the pond's north shore, but the rest require something to float you and your stuff over. This is not Lake George; the waters are not exactly teeming with cabin cruisers. A canoe or kayak should do the trick. Remember, this is primitive camping. There is no potable water source, but picnic tables, fire rings, and pit toilets are provided. With the isolation and the splendid view of Putnam, it's doubtful you'll miss flush toilets or hot showers during your stay.

Even if you haven't reserved an interior site, a boat is certainly worth bringing. There are no restrictions on horsepower, but the pond is ideally suited for small motors and self-propelled crafts. Anglers, who cast for smallmouth bass and tiger muskies, will be pleased, while water-skiers will likely not be. The many ponds in the adjacent Pharaoh Mountain Wilderness offer long stretches of water for canoes, but those who wish to paddle in the remote woods should be prepared to portage at least half a mile to reach their destination.

Landlubbers need not worry. There are plenty of things to do on dry land. Trails to Rock Pond and Treadway Mountain are easily accessible from a parking lot near the campground's boat launch. Many hikers set out on the Long Swing Trail for a day trip to the wonderfully named Grizzle Ocean, or soldier on for a multiday backpack to Pharaoh Lake, Pharaoh Mountain, and beyond. Lean-tos are distributed along the trails, but these are so often occupied that the campground serves

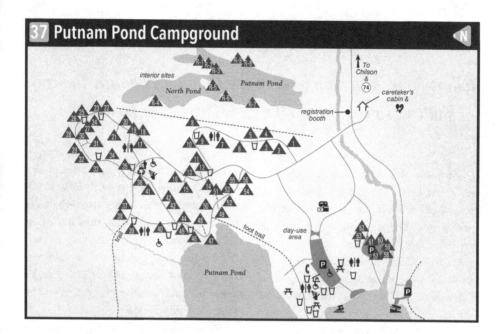

37 Putnam Pond Campground

as overflow for unlucky souls who cannot find a shelter in the backcountry.

Back in Ticonderoga, history buffs can learn about the area's role in the Revolution and in the French and Indian War. If Israel Putnam is to be believed, it was not far from here that he was once captured, tied to a tree, and subjected to a game of William Tell by an overzealous American Indian using a tomahawk instead of a bow and arrow. The only games that modern visitors need to fear are the ubiquitous minigolf courses in nearby Lake George, the largest town in the Adirondacks. If you are like us, you'll prefer to stay close to Putnam Pond and enjoy the surrounding wilderness.

:: Getting There

From I-87 (Adirondack Northway), take Exit 28. Take NY 74 East 12.5 miles. Turn right on CR 39 (Putts Pond Road) and follow it 4 miles to the campground entrance, straight ahead.

GPS COORDINATES   N43° 50.417'   W73° 34.033'

38

Rollins Pond

Rollins Pond, although busy in the summer, is hardly the zoo (or shall we say aquarium?) that is Fish Creek Pond.

Driving by the entrance booth that serves both Fish Creek Pond and Rollins Pond Campgrounds, we were admittedly apprehensive. The first campground of the two, Fish Creek, was packed to the gills with cavalcades of RVs and noisy hordes. Although many sites were along the water, they were badly spaced and bursting at the seams with vehicles of all sorts—not our idea of a peaceful night in the woods. We stayed positive and drove through Fish Creek along the only road to Rollins Pond. The young woman at the registration booth had told us that tent campers prefer Rollins, and we wanted to know why. Short drives to Saranac Lake, Lake Placid, and Tupper Lake make this a great location to start explorations of the High Peaks Wilderness, the St. Regis Canoe Area, and beyond. But whether or not it was truly a hospitable place for those of us who travel light and sleep in tents was still to be determined.

We are happy to report that it is worth a stay. Rollins Pond, while busy in the summer, is hardly the zoo (or shall we say aquarium?) that is Fish Creek Pond. This may be because there are no day-use facilities and no beach manned by lifeguards (Fish Creek serves that purpose). It may also be because there are fewer waterfront sites at Rollins and a restriction on boat-motor size. Or it may be the longer drive—a 10-mile-per-hour slog past almost 200 of Fish Creek's sites—that turns some away. Whatever the reason, it is all a blessing.

While you must pass by the registration booth for Fish Creek to get to Rollins Pond, you will have to check in at a second booth once you reach the second campground. Just past this booth, on the southern side of the pond, you will find the well-spaced waterfront sites of A1–A31, which are some of the nicest in the campground. In general, the best sites are on the southern side of the pond, so it would also be hard to go wrong choosing from sites 1–52, many of which are located directly along the pond's shores (sites 24, 26, 29, 31, 33, 39, 44, 46, and 49 are all off-water sites, but often open onto views of the water). All sites in the campground are shaded by a mix of firs and hardwoods.

The central section of the campground, particularly sites 53–107, is more crowded, and most sites here are located along the edge of a slope that leads down to the water. If you can, choose a site in another section. Farther north along the water, sites in the 140s open onto a small swimming area (though it's not an official beach). With the exception of 102, 103, and 252–257, which are not as private as

:: Ratings

BEAUTY: ★ ★ ★
PRIVACY: ★ ★ ★
QUIET: ★ ★
CLEANLINESS: ★ ★ ★
SECURITY: ★ ★ ★ ★
SPACIOUSNESS: ★ ★ ★

:: Key Information

ADDRESS: 4523 NY 30, Saranac Lake, NY 12983

OPERATED BY: New York State Department of Environmental Conservation

CONTACT: 518-891-3239; www.dec.ny .gov/outdoor/24494.html

OPEN: Mid-May–early September

SITES: 286

SITE AMENITIES: Picnic table and fire ring

ASSIGNMENT: Choose from available sites or reservations

REGISTRATION: On arrival or by reservation

FACILITIES: Water, pit and flush toilets, showers

PARKING: At site, maximum 2 vehicles

FEE: $20/night

ELEVATION: 1,614'

RESTRICTIONS:

- **Pets:** Dogs on leash with proof of currently valid rabies vaccination
- **Fires:** In fire rings only
- **Alcohol:** At site
- **Vehicles:** Up to 40'
- **Other:** Quiet hours 10 p.m.–7 a.m.; 25-horsepower boat-motor restriction
- **Reservations:** 1-night stay allowed

one might wish, almost any site found farther north along the pond is a good choice. When placing a reservation (or if you're a walk-in visitor checking the campground map), it is obvious which sites are off-water.

The pond, which vaguely resembles a sea horse in shape, is large, but that doesn't mean that it's swarming with speedboats. Motors of more than 25 horsepower are prohibited, and the majority of vessels are canoes and kayaks, including rentals available near the boat launch. There is some privately owned land on Rollins, but that does not spoil the lovely views. For even quieter paddling, drop your boat in the smaller Whey Pond, located across the road at the southern end of the campground. No motorboats are permitted on Whey, making it a peaceful place to fish for brook and rainbow trout.

A beach-volleyball court alongside the shower house may keep some amused, but for most activities on dry land, you will have to travel outside the campground. At site 257, the Otter Hollow Loop trail sets out for 1.6 miles to Flood Passage at Floodwood

Pond, and then on for almost 3 more miles to Fish Creek Pond Campground. For longer backcountry treks, hikers can follow trails in all directions to explore the St. Regis Canoe Area. Of course, visitors best appreciate this area by boat, and paddlers may want to use Rollins as a staging point for longer trips.

Lake Placid and its Olympic facilities serve as the biggest draw for tourists in the Adirondacks, and a visit to the top of the ski jump or a drive up Whiteface Mountain can be fun, if not exactly strenuous, activities. Tupper Lake's Wild Center, a museum and miniature zoo designed by the same people who put together the Smithsonian Institution's Air and Space Museum in Washington, D.C., has exhibits featuring local wildlife. Saranac Lake, the closest village to the campground, is a charming place to grab a meal or do a little shopping.

So as not to be misleading, we can tell you there are definitely quieter, more remote, and more scenic facilities to be found in the Adirondacks, but should you be lucky enough to score a waterfront site

38 Rollins Pond Campground

(reservations are strongly recommended), a night or two at Rollins Pond will make for a pleasant getaway. Though this is a very large campground, its website describes it well: "This campground is considered by some as an overflow for Fish Creek Pond Campground, but many have discovered it to be a quiet alternative to its bigger neighbor." We assume you won't be trading in your Kelty, Marmot, or North Face gear anytime soon for a rolling home. As long as Rollins Pond doesn't trade in its wonderful location and its lovely waters, we can forgive it the occasional crowded weekend.

:: Getting There

From I-87 (Adirondack Northway), take Exit 30 to NY 73 North and follow it 28 miles. In Lake Placid, take NY 86 West about 15 miles to CR 186 West, just past Saranac Lake. Pass Adirondack Regional Airport, turn left on NY 30 South, and drive 9 miles to enter Fish Creek Pond Campground. Go to Rollins Pond from site 135.

GPS COORDINATES (FISH CREEK POND CAMPGROUND ENTRANCE)
  N44° 18.367' W74° 24.233'

39

Sacandaga

Campers can be lulled to sleep by the sound of rushing water rather than humming generators.

What is the oldest public campground in the state? It depends on whom you ask. The debate still rages (for lack of a better word) among workers for the Department of Environmental Conservation. In the Catskills, they may tell you it's Devil's Tombstone. In the Adirondacks, they're likely to say it's Sacandaga. It officially became a campground in 1920, but the area had been popular for years with passersby during the time when large stretches of the road did not offer motels. The campground borders the Sacandaga River at the point where its west branch splits off, hence its local nickname "The Forks."

With so many campgrounds in the state located on lakes, it is refreshing to find one on a river. Mind you, this is not like the wide and deep stretches of the Hudson or the Delaware. Although plenty of people will enjoy plopping an inner tube into the Sacandaga's little patches of whitewater, kayakers and canoeists will be disappointed to know that the campground doesn't even have a car-top boat launch,

much less a launch for trailered boats. And when summer comes, the water often dries up, exposing the rocky riverbed. If you have a motorboat, you are better off driving south to where the river empties into Great Sacandaga Lake, a truly impressive reservoir with enough water—nearly 300 billion gallons—to go around. It was created in 1930 when the Sacandaga was dammed to prevent flooding in the region.

The Sacandaga campground also lacks a beach. In the past it had one, but in the 1970s, the Department of Environmental Conservation removed the small dam that collected water and made it deep enough for wading. Because plenty of beaches await within driving distance, it's hardly a tragic loss. Sacandaga remains an attractive campground precisely because it does not cater to day-trippers and RVs full of sunbathers. In sites along the river's edge, campers can be lulled to sleep by the sound of rushing water rather than by humming generators. And since the campground rarely reaches capacity, you do not have to reserve the best sites months in advance.

As you enter the campground, it may not seem promising. Sites 1–6 sit along the river but are crowded together and poorly shaded. Sites 7–60 lie under tall fir trees, but are even more densely packed and, except for 40–44, are essentially out in the open. Better suited for RVs than tents, these sites were completely empty when we

:: Ratings

BEAUTY: ★ ★ ★ ★
PRIVACY: ★ ★ ★
QUIET: ★ ★ ★ ★
CLEANLINESS: ★ ★ ★ ★
SECURITY: ★ ★ ★ ★
SPACIOUSNESS: ★ ★ ★

:: Key Information

ADDRESS: 1047 NY 30, Northville, NY 12134

OPERATED BY: New York State Department of Environmental Conservation

CONTACT: 518-924-4121; www.dec.ny.gov/outdoor/24495.html

OPEN: Mid-May–early October

SITES: 143

SITE AMENITIES: Picnic table and fire ring

ASSIGNMENT: Choose from available sites or reservations

REGISTRATION: On arrival or by reservation

FACILITIES: Water, flush toilets, showers, pay phone

PARKING: At site, maximum 2 vehicles

FEE: $20/night

ELEVATION: 954'

RESTRICTIONS:

▓ **Pets:** Dogs on leash with proof of currently valid rabies vaccination

▓ **Fires:** In fire rings only

▓ **Alcohol:** At site

▓ **Vehicles:** Up to 30'

▓ **Other:** Quiet hours 10 p.m.–7 a.m.

▓ **Reservations:** 2-night stay required

visited, and for good reason. This is essentially an overflow area, and you should not bother reserving them.

Instead, choose something at either "The Island" or "The Berry Patch." Named by the campground staff years ago, The Island (sites 61–119) is located at the fork of the Sacandaga and its west branch. A sturdy, narrow bridge over the river leads to these sites from the day-use area at the northern end of the campground. Many are tempted to book site 62 or 64, and those are certainly good choices. Tent campers wishing for more room, however, would be wise to go with site 96 or 97, in the northwest corner of the campground. These two sites require parking along the road and walking about 20–30 yards down to spacious clearings along the West Branch. In general, we've found the sites along the West Branch to be the most desirable, but any site along the water will make for an enjoyable stay. Interior sites are well shaded by a mix of firs and hardwoods and provide easy access to the two comfort stations—but they are

no different from any other standard site you may find in the Adirondacks.

The Berry Patch (sites 120–144) was named for all the wild berries that grow on the southern end of the campground. In the past, the berries have been known to attract a black bear or two. As in most parts of the Adirondacks, bears are a concern here, and you should heed the campground's precautions, but it is unlikely that you will ever see one. The Berry Patch should be a little quieter than The Island. Under the shade of tall fir trees, it is a scenic patch of sites, but the spaces themselves are a bit more jumbled together. The best of the bunch is 123, which is spacious and well situated along the river.

Even though so many sites provide easy access to the riverbank, swimming is at your own risk. Anglers come for the trout (brook, brown, and rainbow). Families with kids will appreciate the campground's Junior Naturalist program. Although no trails depart directly from the campground, the 133-mile Northville–Placid Trail has a terminus along Route 30, on the western end of a

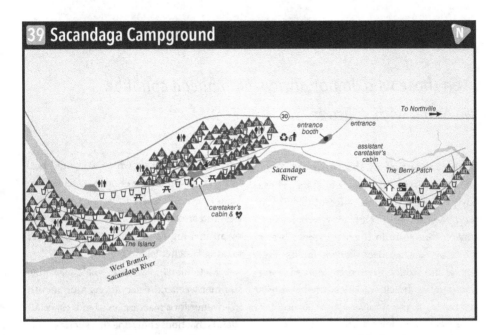

39 Sacandaga Campground

bridge over the Sacandaga. For 10 miles the trail follows NY 30, a major road running north–south through the Adirondacks, and only those trying to complete all 133 miles feel the need to hike this section. If you are looking for an easy day hike, try the 3-mile round-trip trek to Auger Falls, 10 miles north of the campground, off NY 30.

Quiet, safe, and easily accessible, Sacandaga has been a family favorite for generations. Many retirees have been coming to the campground since they were children. They return every year, some even staying the entire summer, shuffling spots once every two weeks. If that is not an endorsement, we don't know what is.

:: Getting There

From I-90 (New York State Thruway), take Exit 27, Amsterdam, to NY 30 North and follow it about 40 miles. The campground is on the left.

GPS COORDINATES   N43°21.417'   W74°16.950'

40

Saranac Lake Islands

Even those who do not always plan ahead could be rewarded with solitude.

In the language of the Iroquois, *Saranac* is said to mean "cluster of stars." These days, the word conjures different feelings in most New Yorkers. Nearly every grocery and convenience store in the state stocks brews made by Saranac Beer, known for its ales, lagers, and stouts. Brewed by Matt Brewing Company in the city of Utica, the beverages are made, as the website claims, from "the pure water that flows from the Adirondacks and the grains that grow in its unspoiled soil." Saranac Lakes, a charming village west of Lake Placid, does nothing to sully the brewery's reputation. Its three lakes (Upper, Middle, and Lower) are among the mountains' most beautiful.

Campers who own boats or are willing to spend a little money on a rental should put this book down now and reserve a campsite on Lower or Middle Saranac Lakes. With 87 primitive sites (including three with lean-tos) to choose from along the shores and on the islands of the two lakes, you are guaranteed an unforgettable Adirondack camping experience. We explored the lakes in our

:: Ratings

BEAUTY: ★ ★ ★ ★ ★
PRIVACY: ★ ★ ★ ★ ★
QUIET: ★ ★ ★ ★ ★
CLEANLINESS: ★ ★ ★ ★
SECURITY: ★ ★ ★ ★
SPACIOUSNESS: ★ ★ ★ ★ ★

$100 inflatable kayak, which we would hesitate to take out on the choppy waters of, say, Lake George. It was perfect for these beauties, and after a good paddle we were greeted by an inviting campsite upon a ridge overlooking Hatchet Island.

Meticulous planners will make their summer weekend reservations nine months in advance for a place on an island, especially islands that house only one site, such as Green (13), Coal Pit (22), Larom (23), Partridge (24), Goose (27), Duck (28), Hocum Point (35), Shaw (71), Norway (74), Bartlett (75), Halfway (77), and Tick (84). As desirable as these sites are, they are not all that different from shoreline sites. The wilderness is thick, there are no hiking trails, and development is prohibited on both Lower and Middle Saranac Lakes. Consequently, every site is isolated, and when the sun sets, campers along the shorelines may as well be on an island.

The majority of sites are located on Lower Saranac Lake (1–62), and all are easily reached by motorboat. Paddlers will have to do a little work to get out to the Narrows and Loon Bay on the west side of the lake. Arrive early if you plan to camp at sites 45–47, especially if you need to make multiple trips to ferry your supplies. Lower Saranac can be accessed from the State Bridge Boat Launch along NY 3. Boaters put in at Second Pond, where only one site (number 62) is found. For all other sites, campers must make their way under the State Bridge (NY 3) and into

:: Key Information

ADDRESS: 4468 State Route 3, Saranac Lake, NY 12983

OPERATED BY: New York State Department of Environmental Conservation

CONTACT: 518-891-2841; www.dec.ny.gov/outdoor/24496.html

OPEN: Mid-May–early October

SITES: 87

SITE AMENITIES: Picnic table and fire ring

ASSIGNMENT: Choose from available sites or reservations

REGISTRATION: On arrival or by reservation

FACILITIES: Pit toilets

PARKING: Limited at State Bridge boat launch, near registration booth

FEE: $22/night

ELEVATION: 1,541'

RESTRICTIONS:

■ **Pets:** Dogs on leash with proof of currently valid rabies vaccination

■ **Fires:** In fire rings only

■ **Alcohol:** At site

■ **Vehicles:** None permitted; sites are accessible only by boat.

■ **Other:** Quiet hours 10 p.m.–7 a.m.; carry out all trash

■ **Reservations:** 1-night stay allowed

First Pond, also home to just one site, number 61. Others must follow the channel markers through a narrow passage to the southern end of Lower Saranac and the rest of the sites on the lake.

A campground map is needed to locate all of the sites. The scale of the lake can be overwhelming, and with many bays and islands to explore, it is easy to get confused. Signs designating sites are not always easy to see, especially in the evening. A less-popular car-top boat launch and a comfort station are on the eastern end of the lake in Ampersand Bay. Day visitors often use this launch to access Eagle Island (sites 1–5), designated as a day-use area for picnickers.

The sites on Middle Saranac Lake (63–87) are even more remote and therefore attract more campers with canoes or kayaks looking for quiet. Although the development of the campground at Lower Saranac officially began in 1934, the sites on Middle Saranac were not added until 1992. The lake remains an unspoiled delight, with isolated beaches and dunes along the shoreline. It is

possible to launch a boat from State Bridge and enter Middle Saranac through Kelly Slough on the western end of Lower Saranac. Traveling this way, you will navigate the Saranac River and pass through a set of hand-operated locks, a lovely trip if you are not in a rush. If time is a factor, drive 4 miles west along Route 3 from State Bridge to a parking lot and put in at South Creek on the southern end of Middle Saranac.

On the northern end of Middle Saranac, tiny Weller Pond is a haven for paddlers with tents. Motorboats turn back at the narrow passage leading to sites 83–87, so this is by far the quietest corner of the campground. Site 87 includes a lean-to, and people tend to reserve it first.

Although many stay here for the full two weeks allowed, others use the campground as a launching pad for longer trips. From Lower Saranac and Second Pond, the Saranac River runs through another set of locks and into Oseetah Lake and Lake Flower, which borders the village of Saranac Lake. From Weller Pond, a portage of about a mile will bring you to Saginaw Bay on the northern end of Upper Saranac Lake. Or a paddle through Bartletts Carry on the southwestern end of Middle Saranac will bring you to the southeastern end of Upper Saranac. The campground doesn't include Upper Saranac because it is open for private development, but it is a magnificent, hourglass-shaped lake that makes up the southern end of the celebrated St. Regis Canoe Area. For a true adventure, the Northern Forest Canoe Trail, which has a terminus in Old Forge, runs through each of the Saranac Lakes and all the way to Fort Kent in Maine. This 740-mile trip awaits experienced, strong-shouldered paddlers and is often referred to as the water version of the Appalachian Trail.

:: Getting There

From I-87 (Adirondack Northway), take Exit 30 to NY 73 North and follow it 28 miles. In Lake Placid, take NY 86 West 9 miles to the village of Saranac Lake. In Saranac Lake, take NY 3 West 6 miles to the State Bridge Boat Launch, on your left.

GPS COORDINATES (STATE BRIDGE BOAT LAUNCH)   N44° 17.283'   W74° 11.117'

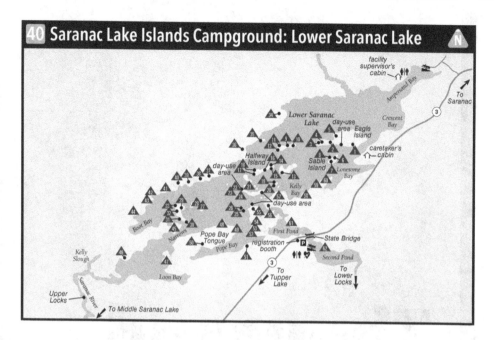

40 Saranac Lake Islands Campground: Lower Saranac Lake

40 Saranac Lake Islands Campground: Middle Saranac Lake

Thousand Islands

41

Mary Island State Park

Mary Island's heavily wooded 12 acres offer the ideal setting in which to enjoy the beauty of the St. Lawrence River.

Along the northern border of New York runs the St. Lawrence River, which flows from Lake Ontario through Canada and finally empties into the Atlantic Ocean. As the river flows more than 800 miles to the Atlantic, it passes a 50-mile stretch filled with more than 1,800 islands. These islands range from roughly 48 square miles to several square feet and, along with more than 3,000 shoals, make the river a veritable maze. Navigating this maze are Jet Skis, powerboats, sailboats, cruise boats, yachts, and even ocean liners, though these behemoths remain within the shipping lanes. Nestled within this maze is Mary Island, a heavily wooded 12 acres that offer the ideal setting in which to enjoy the beauty of the St. Lawrence.

The 12 sites on the island vary widely in size, views, and proximity to the access trails, numerous docks, and each other. The island is oblong, with its main axis running from southwest, where the park office and day-use area are located, to the northeast, a very short distance to Canadian waters.

:: Ratings

BEAUTY: ★ ★ ★ ★ ★
PRIVACY: ★ ★ ★ ★
QUIET: ★ ★ ★ ★
CLEANLINESS: ★ ★
SECURITY: ★ ★ ★ ★ ★
SPACIOUSNESS: ★ ★ ★ ★ ★

Most campers will approach the island from the southwest and initially encounter a service dock, public dock, and a floating campers' dock. You will want to use the middle public dock to register and then move your boat to the neighboring floating dock for sites 1–5, to the northeast floating dock for sites 9–12, or to the sheltered fixed dock on the northeast shore for sites 6–10 (sites 9 and 10 are about equidistant from both northern docks). Alternatively, you can dock at the southeastern tip and access the sites along the central trail or the western trail, though this last trail runs precariously close to some cliffs. The sole comfort station is located roughly in the center of the southeastern half of the island, but it is a short distance to any of the sites.

Site 1 is closest to the office and picnic area, along the eastern edge of the island's southern tip. Although it has great views of the St. Lawrence, campers should be aware that the path to sites 2–4 passes through the site. These last three sites lie among large, exposed slabs of granite and are closely clustered together. Site 2, although exposed, is closest to water and the southeastern campers' dock. Sites 3 and 4 are set back from the shore and have ample shade from cedars, pines, and hardwoods. Considering the proximity of these sites to each other, this area would serve groups better than campers seeking a more solitary experience.

:: Key Information

ADDRESS: 36661 Cedar Point State Park Dr., Clayton, NY 13624

OPERATED BY: New York State Office of Parks, Recreation and Historic Preservation

CONTACT: 315-654-2522; nysparks .com/parks/40/details.aspx

OPEN: Memorial Day–Labor Day

SITES: 12 tent sites

SITE AMENITIES: Picnic table, stand-up grill, and fire ring

ASSIGNMENT: Upon arrival and registration

REGISTRATION: 3 p.m.–9 p.m.

FACILITIES: Picnic areas, potable water, flush toilets, docks

PARKING: At Keewaydin State Park

FEE: $16/night most tent sites (extra $4/ night on Fridays, Saturdays, and holidays)

ELEVATION: 241'

RESTRICTIONS:

■ **Pets:** Dogs on leash with proof of currently valid rabies vaccination

■ **Fires:** In fire rings only

■ **Alcohol:** Allowed

■ **Vehicles:** None permitted; sites are accessible only by boat.

■ **Other:** Quiet hours 10 p.m.–7 a.m.

■ **Reservations:** Not site-specific when reserved online; 2-night stay required; 1-night reservations available if reserved within 3 days of visit

Site 5, which is very spacious, is also on the southern tip but lies on the western shore and is consequently farther from any of the campers' docks. This site is heavily shaded by pines and cedars but has hardly any view of the river because of trees and a small electric-transfer building.

Near site 5 begins the western trail, which you could use to access site 6. However, this portion of the trail passes the precarious cliffs and site 6 can be easily reached from the main trail or the other docks. Site 6 sits high along the western cliffs but they are less precarious here, and the elevation provides expansive views of the river. A thick canopy of pines shades the spacious site, but exposed roots limit the places to pitch a tent.

Site 7 is centrally located and has direct access to the northwest fixed dock. Atop a heavily forested hill, the site offers good views of the river through the surrounding trees. You'll find lots of room to spread out and numerous places to pitch a tent. A short distance north from the docks is site 8, which is undoubtedly the most spacious site on the island. Tall hardwoods shade the area, and numerous patches of grass make ideal places to pitch a tent. The site is also enhanced by great views of the river, though multiple trails serving the next two sites pass either through or very near the site.

At the very northern tip of the island lies site 9, which is one of the most scenic and secluded sites. With panoramic views of the river in three directions, it is hard to not look out to the St. Lawrence. The rugged terrain features exposed bedrock and twisted trees with ample room to spread out on grassy patches of ground. Although some spots are very close to the water, we suspect campers will seek shelter rather than proximity to the water. The wind gusts strongly here, and going fishing for your tent will ruin any trip.

Traveling south along the eastern edge, campers find another great choice at site 10. Sitting atop a small hill, and with plenty of

41 Mary Island State Park Campground

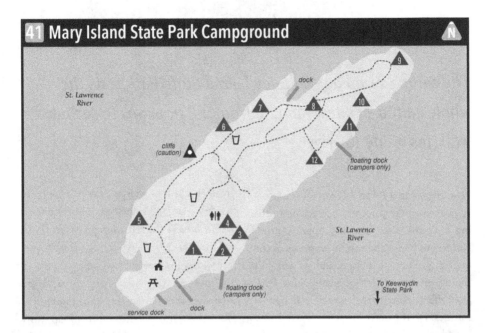

Though Mary Island is only a stone's throw from the tip of Wellesley Island (see next page), the latter area is private. Consequently, the best access point is Keewaydin State Park, about 2 miles away on the mainland. Campers can park vehicles and rent small motorboats here, making Mary Island one of the most convenient boat-only sites in New York. Note that online reservations are not site-specific and sites will be assigned when you register. However, calling before you arrive or reserving by phone will give you a better chance of getting a specific site.

shade from the mixed hardwoods, the site offers views of the river to the east and west, along with plenty of room—large, grassy areas intermingle with exposed bedrock.

The island's remaining two sites are on its northeastern edge near the other floating campers' dock. Site 11 is closest to the dock. Since this site is on the riverbank, there is little shade, but grassy areas offer ample space to set up a tent. Site 12 has several advantages to consider over site 11: it is more spacious, better shaded, and more remote-feeling. Both sites have spectacular views.

:: Getting There

To Keewaydin State Park: From I-81 North, take Exit 50N, NY 12/Alexandria Bay. Continue on NY 12 for 3.2 miles; the park entrance is on the left.

GPS COORDINATES (PARK ENTRANCE)   N44° 21.933'   W75° 55.933'

GPS COORDINATES (SOUTH DOCK)   N44° 21.933'   W75° 55.283'

42

Wellesley Island State Park

The campground at Wellesley Island State Park runs the whole gamut of sites, ranging from full hookups to secluded walk-ins along the river.

The Thousand Islands region is a boater's haven where you can find excellent fishing and unlimited cruising opportunities. Numerous parks and public launches in the region give access to beautiful waters, but the 2,636-acre Wellesley Island State Park also offers many more recreational opportunities. On the northwest edge of Wellesley Island, the park has miles of hiking trails, a sandy swimming beach, a nature center, a golf course, numerous playgrounds and playfields, several boat launches, a recreation center, and a variety of habitats that provide excellent wildlife-viewing. The island can be reached by boat or by driving over the first section of the multiple-span Thousand Islands Bridge, which from the north side of the island crosses the United States border into Canada.

The campground at Wellesley Island State Park runs the gamut of sites, ranging from full hookups to secluded walk-ins along the river. Tent campers should simply ignore

Areas H and F as well as Area C, which are clearly for large RVs. Instead, they should try to find sites in the remaining areas (A, B, D, and E), although the type and quality of sites vary widely in these areas as well.

Most of the sites along Area E are lawn sites that border the surrounding forest. Although most sites on this loop won't please campers who seek beauty and solitude, there are exceptions. One such area (sites 52–56 as well as walk-in site 101) is accessed along a rough spur road—the area juts out into the river slightly, and this provides beautiful views. Large protrusions of bedrock and windswept trees add some privacy while shading the area. However, these small sites are close together and have limited parking. A similar setting exists for sites 61–64 and 66, which share access from a short driveway. Another group of sites, 75–80, has views of the river, although the view consists mostly of a boat launch and docks.

Area A's layout is a mishmash of loops, spurs, and switchbacks, which could make finding your site an adventure. Generally, the sites are grassy, with a few large shade trees along the edges or intermixed. With the exception of sites 17–30, which lie along a hillside with few flat spaces, most sites are spacious. Of particular interest are the wonderful vistas from riverside sites 44–49, which are shielded from the rest of the area by a hill

:: Ratings

BEAUTY: ★ ★ ★ ★
PRIVACY: ★ ★ ★
QUIET: ★ ★
CLEANLINESS: ★ ★ ★
SECURITY: ★ ★ ★
SPACIOUSNESS: ★ ★

:: Key Information

ADDRESS: 44927 Cross Island Rd., Fineview, NY 13640

OPERATED BY: New York State Office of Parks, Recreation and Historic Preservation

CONTACT: 315-482-2722; nysparks .com/parks/52/details.aspx

OPEN: May-mid-October

SITES: 435 tent sites, including 115 electric sites and 57 sites with full hookups

SITE AMENITIES: Picnic table and fire ring

ASSIGNMENT: Choose from available sites or reservations

REGISTRATION: 3 p.m.-9 p.m.

FACILITIES: Picnic areas, potable water, flush toilets, boat launch, showers, marina, 9-hole golf course

PARKING: At site or in designated area near carry-in sites

FEE: $15/night most tent sites; $21 waterfront sites

ELEVATION: 253'

RESTRICTIONS:

■ **Pets:** Dogs on leash with proof of currently valid rabies vaccination

■ **Fires:** In fire rings only

■ **Alcohol:** Allowed

■ **Vehicles:** RVs limited to specific sites

■ **Other:** Quiet hours 10 p.m.-7 a.m.

■ **Reservations:** 2-night stay required; 1-night reservations available if reserved within 3 days of visit

and feel more isolated. These sites are shallow, close together, and dense with trees, precluding large trailers or RVs. A similar group of shady sites (56, 58, and 60–62) lies ahead on the road. This group has views of the river, but, lacking a hill, is not as private.

As with Area A, Area D has some sites that are grassy with few shade trees. The sites here are well sized, except for sites 1–7, which are particularly small and public. The prime sites (9–12, 14, 15, 19, and 20) have shade, privacy, and stunning views of the river. Although these sites are definitely a good choice, tent campers should also consider the excellent walk-in sites, 26–28. Access and parking for these sites are beyond site 29, down a hill toward Area B, and on a lawn to the right. A short walk over a small hill to the riverbank reveals spacious, shady sites with panoramic views of the river.

Whereas most areas here have only a few gems mixed with a majority of

less-desirable sites, Area B is just the opposite. The entire area feels secluded, and sites seem to grow out of the woods rather than encircle large communal lawns. In general, the sites on the river side of the road are hidden away among the trees, while those on the opposite side are visible from the road and lack views. When making reservations, campers should be aware that sites 26–32 are electric and intended for RVs. Also, a high-traffic area exists at the end of the area where Areas B and C come together and exit through Area A.

Those disclaimers aside, the campground's designated prime sites (1, 2, 6–8, 14–23, 34–39, and 42) are excellent, have sufficient space, ample shade, and exceptional views of the river. Sites 1 and 2 share access and lie downhill from the road where it climbs toward the rest of the area. Consequently, these sites feel more remote and are a great choice, since they lie directly on

42 Wellesley Island State Park Campground: Areas A–D

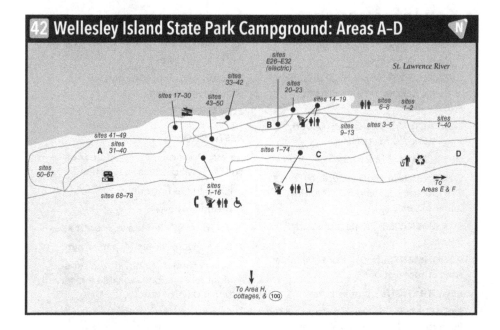

the riverfront. Access to sites 6–8 is via a rugged dirt road with blind corners that makes a steep descent toward the river. It has no turnaround, so you may want to walk this spur road to plan your entrance and exit. Site 8 sits above the river and closer to the main road, whereas sites 6 and 7 are right on the riverbank and basically blend together. A little farther away is a grassy parking area for walk-in sites 14–19—campers must climb over a steep wooded knoll to access these. Situated above the St. Lawrence River on a granite outcrop, the sites serve as a retreat from the bustle of the rest of the campground. The remaining prime sites (20–23, 34–39, and 42) sit right on the riverbank, grouped in bunches of twos and threes and reached by rough, narrow roads.

:: Getting There

From I-81 North, cross over the Thousand Islands Bridge and take Exit 51, Island Road/Island Parks. Turn right on CR 191 and follow it 0.5 mile. Turn right on Thousand Islands Park Road/CR 100. After 0.5 mile, turn right on Cross Island Road and follow it to the park entrance.

GPS COORDINATES   N44° 19.000'   W76° 01.250'

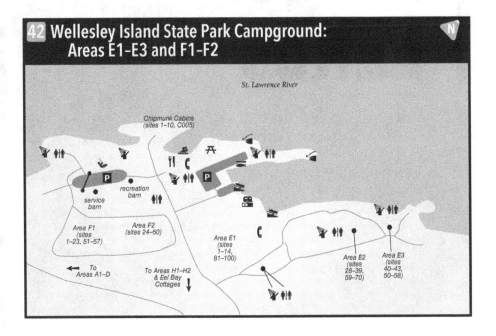

Finger
Lakes

43

Buttermilk Falls State Park

The idea of a campground practically inside a city may seem
strange to some, but not if you know Ithaca.

On the very edge of Ithaca's southern boundary lies a multiuse park that offers a special opportunity for campers wishing to visit this unique Finger Lakes city. The idea of a campground practically inside a city may seem strange to some, but not if you know Ithaca. Located on the southern tip of Cayuga Lake, Ithaca presents outdoors enthusiasts with numerous activities as well as access to a wide variety of restaurants, bustling nightlife, and nearby wine trails. Ithaca seems to be surrounded by nature—in fact, there are four state parks along with numerous city- and university-managed parks within the immediate vicinity. Given the wide variety of outdoor activities available here, Buttermilk Falls State Park serves as an ideal base to explore the region.

The park includes Lake Treman and a wetland, as well as the gorge that surrounds Buttermilk Creek. Each of these natural features can be explored along short hiking trails, though the gorge is the park's most astounding natural feature and obviously its most popular attraction. The gorge and its

:: Ratings

BEAUTY: ★ ★
PRIVACY: ★ ★ ★
QUIET: ★ ★ ★
CLEANLINESS: ★ ★ ★
SECURITY: ★ ★ ★
SPACIOUSNESS: ★ ★

striking, deep pools were dramatically carved by Buttermilk Creek, which drops from 1,000 feet to 400 feet above sea level. The water's sculpting power is particularly evident at Pinnacle Rock, a tall spire near the end of the Gorge Trail. This trail, as you might suspect, winds through the gorge, often sharing the creek bed and taking you past stone walls and up stone staircases. The stone work, originally built by the Civilian Conservation Corps during the Depression, provides an interesting comparison of man's and nature's work on the local stone. At Buttermilk Falls, the creek cascades white and frothy across a wide rock face and tumbles to a pool below. At the base of this waterfall, a small but deep swimming area is accessible by the park's lower entrance and main parking lot.

You can reach the park's campground from this same parking area. It is separated from the rest of the park by a long, winding paved road that climbs a steep hillside. The camping area, which begins with a handful of rental cabins, is laid out in a single loop with a short spur road containing four more tent sites. All of the sites, which are mostly dirt with some grassy spots, are shaded by a canopy of mixed hardwood trees. Without much understory, the sites are visible to each other. But they're amply spaced, and changes in elevation between the area's eastern and western edges prevent it from feeling crowded.

The sites along the western edge lie near a drop-off and have less space

:: Key Information

ADDRESS: NY 13, Ithaca, NY 14850

OPERATED BY: New York State Office of Parks, Recreation and Historic Preservation

CONTACT: 607-273-5761; nysparks .com/parks/151/details.aspx

OPEN: Early May–Early October

SITES: 45

SITE AMENITIES: Picnic table and fire ring

ASSIGNMENT: Choose from available sites or reservations

REGISTRATION: 3 p.m.–9 p.m.

FACILITIES: Picnic areas, pavilions, playground, swimming area, bathhouse, potable water, flush toilets, showers

PARKING: At site

FEE: $15/night (plus $4/night on Fridays, Saturdays, and holidays)

ELEVATION: 410'

RESTRICTIONS:

■ **Pets:** Dogs on leash with proof of currently valid rabies vaccination

■ **Fires:** In fire rings only

■ **Alcohol:** Prohibited in swimming area

■ **Vehicles:** RVs and trailers allowed

■ **Other:** Quiet hours 10 p.m.–7 a.m.; 6 people maximum/site; maximum 14-night stay

■ **Reservations:** 2-night stay required

than those on the interior of the loop. The sites on the eastern outer edge are the most desirable: spacious and private, they border the surrounding woods. The four sites situated along a short spur road at the end of the campground loop provide the most privacy.

Campers who can't find a site at Buttermilk Falls can drive south a little over 1 mile to Robert H. Treman State Park, where there are considerably more campsites. However, a grassy field hosts most of the sites here, and they offer little in the way of shade or privacy. From this state park, adventurers can hike along Enfield Creek and its related gorge, which has waterfalls and water-sculpted rocks.

Fillmore Glen State Park, a short drive north of Ithaca, offers more hiking trails in another dramatic gorge. You can camp here as well, though the sites are even more crowded and less private than the ones at Robert H. Treman State Park.

Boaters wishing to gain access to Cayuga Lake can drive north from Buttermilk Falls State Park a few miles to Allan H. Treman State Marine Park, where there is a boat launch, or about 15 miles farther to Taughannock Falls State Park (see its description on page 158). Since access to one state park grants vehicle access to others on the same day, take the time to explore the trails and gorges at these other parks as well. After all, as the saying goes, "Ithaca is gorges."

43 Buttermilk Falls State Park Campground

:: Getting There

From I-81 South, take Exit 12, NY 281/Cortland. Stay left on the exit ramp until you reach the stop sign. Turn left onto NY 281 and follow it 3.8 miles. NY 281 becomes NY 13; continue on NY 13 for 21 miles through Dryden into Ithaca. After passing NY 79/Main Street, continue 2 miles; the park entrance is on the left.

GPS COORDINATES   N42° 25.033'   W76° 31.300'

44

Keuka Lake State Park

Shaped like a Y, Keuka Lake is sometimes called Crooked Lake.

A bird's-eye view of western New York reveals 11 narrow lakes, each of which runs roughly north–south. Their unusual likenesses to fingers on a hand obviously led to their name, the Finger Lakes. Keuka Lake is the only lake among the 11 that is not perfectly linear in shape: it is shaped like a *Y* and so is sometimes called Crooked Lake. Further, the lake is distinct from its neighbors in that it is also the only one that drains into another of the Finger Lakes—in this case, into Seneca Lake by way of Keuka Lake Outlet. At one time, this outlet was transformed into a canal that connected the two lakes, but it was eventually abandoned as a canal in 1877. Aside from these characteristics, it shares all of the other familiar traits of a Finger Lake in that it is glacially formed, is very deep, has its own wine trail, and is an ideal place to go fishing or boating. Incidentally, Keuka comes from the Iroquois word *kyoo-ka*, which means "canoe landing."

The campground at Keuka Lake lies uphill from the park entrance. Laid out in three large, one-way loops— Deer Run, Twin Fawns, and Esperanza View—the sites are spacious, open to the sky, grassy, and spread out along the loops. Dense stands of conifers in the center of each loop effectively divide the loop into smaller, private sections. Most sites claim a shade tree as well as shrubs and thick vegetation, which increases privacy. The sites are large enough for a camping area, vehicles, and a small boat trailer. Considering that the lake is the park's main feature, space for a boat is a great benefit. A comfort station and playground serve each loop. Dumpsters and recycling stations are situated along the access road.

The Deer Run Loop (sites 51–100) is a little less private than the other loops, but has many good sites. None of the sites in this loop contain electric hookups. You'll find the best sites along the beginning of the loop, on the eastern edge and interior. These sites have dense shrubs and grasses as well as large shade trees. Where the loop turns back toward the entrance, the sites become more open, with less shade and vegetation, making them less private. Near the loop's entrance, the sites become wide open, with no shade and only sparse vegetation. The exterior campsites are clearly visible from the access road; the interior campsites have direct access to the playground.

The Twin Fawns Loop (sites 1–50) contains the park's most shady sites, graced as they are by very large willows. The loop's exterior contains the shadiest sites as well as denser vegetation serving as dividers. The best sites, both on the interior and exterior,

:: Ratings

BEAUTY: ★ ★
PRIVACY: ★ ★ ★ ★
QUIET: ★ ★ ★
CLEANLINESS: ★ ★ ★ ★
SECURITY: ★ ★ ★
SPACIOUSNESS: ★ ★ ★ ★ ★

:: Key Information

ADDRESS: 3560 Pepper Rd., Bluff Point, NY 14478

OPERATED BY: New York State Office of Parks, Recreation and Historic Preservation

CONTACT: 315-536-3666; nysparks.com/parks/67/details.aspx

OPEN: Early May–mid-October

SITES: 150 tent sites, including 53 electric sites

SITE AMENITIES: Picnic table and fire ring

ASSIGNMENT: Choose from available sites or reservations

REGISTRATION: 3 p.m.–9 p.m.

FACILITIES: Picnic areas, pavilion, potable water, flush toilets, boat launch, showers

PARKING: At site

FEE: $15/night most tent sites (plus $4/night on Fridays, Saturdays, and holidays)

ELEVATION: 817'

RESTRICTIONS:

■ **Pets:** Dogs on leash with proof of currently valid rabies vaccination

■ **Fires:** In fire rings only

■ **Alcohol:** Allowed

■ **Vehicles:** RVs and trailers allowed

■ **Other:** Quiet hours 10 p.m.–7 a.m.

■ **Reservations:** 2-night stay required

lie on the loop's western edge and are primarily nonelectric. Farther along the loop, the sites are quite large and most have electric hookups. Unlike the Deer Run Loop, all of the sites here are effectively removed from the rest of the sites within the loop, making them a little more desirable.

The last loop, Esperanza View (101–150), consists of an upper section along its eastern edge and a lower section on its western edge. The change in elevation and a dense conifer center increase this loop's overall privacy, but sites in the upper section are far more desirable than those in the lower section. There are fewer shade trees in the upper section, but this permits views up and down the lake valley. Sites in the upper section, though almost entirely electric, offer added privacy with an additional border of dense shrubs along the roadside. The configuration of shrubs and trees creates the feeling of outdoor rooms.

Campers won't find as many hiking opportunities here as at some other New York campgrounds, but access to the lake and its related water sports are the real attraction. The lake is the third largest of the Finger Lakes: its width varies from 0.5 mile to 2 miles along its 19.6-mile length. The total surface area measures roughly 11,730 acres, and the deepest point is 183 feet. Visitors can use the public boat launch, located past the park's picnic and swimming areas, after paying the park entrance fee. Boating and fishing regulations are available at the entrance and on the web at **keukalakeassoc.org**. Diving, motorboats, Jet Skis, and waterskiing are all allowed, as are sailboats, kayaks, and canoes.

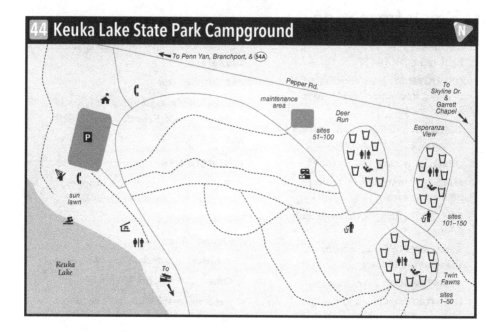

:: Getting There

From I-90 (New York State Thruway), take Exit 42. Take NY 14 South through Geneva; 12.7 miles past Geneva, bear right on NY 54. Turn right to stay on NY 54 and go 4.5 miles to Penn Yan. Go left on NY 54/Main Street, then right on NY 54A/Elm Street. Follow NY 54A 6.3 miles, then go left on Pepper Road. The park entrance is on the right.

GPS COORDINATES   N42° 35.450'   W77° 07.833'

45

Stony Brook State Park

*Few of the Finger Lakes region's parks offer as scenic
a campground as the one at Stony Brook.*

The Finger Lakes region was shaped by multiple periods of glaciation during the Ice Age. Indeed, the entire state of New York, except in the region of Allegany State Park, bears the scars and deposits of huge sheets of ice. The most striking of the glacial effects, other than the region's lakes, are the dramatic gorges that formed as the last sheets of ice receded from the region. Long swaths through hillsides were eroded further as brooks and streams cut away the softer sedimentary rock. These gorges can be seen throughout the region, but no state park other than Stony Brook allows you to camp along the water's edge. Although Stony Brook's camping areas are not situated within the most dramatic parts of the gorge, you can choose among plenty of scenic brook-side sites.

The park's campground is divided into two areas, the first of which contains sites 1–53 and is laid out as a single loop with one spur road. Large evergreens provide ample shade throughout this area, though the trees are densest at the exterior of the loop and

along the spur road. Along the southern edge of the loop and spur is a steep hillside, at the bottom of which flows a stream that feeds Stony Brook. Sites that back up to this edge look down upon the stream and into the surrounding forest. Sites on the loop's interior are close together, grassy, and very public due to proximity to this area's comfort station. The first few sites (16–19) on the loop's exterior are also grassy but very small, as they back up to a hillside that separates them from ones on the spur road. The other sites along the exterior of the loop are larger and have a gravelly dirt base. The spur road rises above the loop sites, which effectively removes sites along the spur road (35–53) from the more public spaces of this area. These sites are more densely wooded and have a gravelly dirt base as well. Most sites along the spur road are grouped in threes or fours that share narrow parking areas. This configuration makes it hard to tell where some sites begin and end. Consequently, these grouped sites are probably best suited to large camping parties— solitary campers would likely prefer some of the other sites this park has to offer.

The second area, sites 54–130, is by far the largest, with some spacious sites along Stony Brook. Like those in the previous area, these sites are shaded by large evergreens, and the trees here are denser than those at the sites mentioned above. Similarly, these sites also have gravelly dirt bases with no shrubbery or understory. The layout

:: Ratings

BEAUTY: ★ ★ ★ ★
PRIVACY: ★ ★ ★
QUIET: ★ ★ ★
CLEANLINESS: ★ ★ ★
SECURITY: ★ ★ ★
SPACIOUSNESS: ★ ★ ★

:: Key Information

ADDRESS: 10820 Route 36S, Dansville, NY 14437

OPERATED BY: New York State Office of Parks, Recreation and Historic Preservation

CONTACT: 585-335-8111; nysparks .com/parks/118/details.aspx

OPEN: Early May–early October

SITES: 119 tent sites

SITE AMENITIES: Picnic table and fire ring

ASSIGNMENT: Choose from available sites or reservations

REGISTRATION: 3 p.m.–9 p.m.

FACILITIES: Picnic areas, pavilion, potable water, flush toilets, concession stand, bathhouse, tennis courts, playground, showers

PARKING: At site

FEE: $15/night most tent sites; $19/night prime tent sites (plus $4/night on Fridays, Saturdays, and holidays)

ELEVATION: 384'

RESTRICTIONS:

■ **Pets:** Dogs on leash with proof of currently valid rabies vaccination

■ **Fires:** In fire rings only

■ **Alcohol:** Not allowed in campground

■ **Vehicles:** RVs and trailers allowed

■ **Other:** Quiet hours 10 p.m.–8 a.m.

■ **Reservations:** 2-night stay required

includes a very small loop and a much larger loop consisting of both an upper and lower leg. Where the upper and lower legs reconnect, a short road to a public parking area begins. This layout allows the sites to feel removed from the entire campground but not from their immediate neighbors. As campers descend from the park's main road to this area and its upper leg, they will see the very small loop of congested sites (55–60). Near this small loop are several more shared-access sites (54 and 68–72). Along the outer edge of the upper leg, you'll find many large sites with features similar to most other sites in this area.

Down at the lower leg, the interior sites back up to the hillside that separates the upper and lower legs, and thus have a more enclosed feel. These sites are well spaced, with some being deep and large. The first few sites (112–116) on the lower leg's exterior are set back from the road toward Stony Brook—these sites share the same parking area. The remaining sites along the exterior of the leg lie directly on the edge of Stony Brook, which makes these sites unique to the campground. Sites along the water's edge are not as spacious as some of the others, but there are a few gems. As you drive back up to the upper leg, you find the park's remaining sites (87–92)—these are very small, grassy sites wedged between the road and a steep hillside.

The park has three hiking trails, two along the gorge's rim and one along the gorge's bottom, all of which are accessible from the campground area. The three trails join at the lower end of the gorge, where a dam across the brook previously provided the park's swimming area. As of 2012, the swimming area is closed, though campers may use the swimming area at Letchworth State Park (see page 172 for its description). Admission to Letchworth Park is free with your camping permit, but you'll pay an additional fee to use the pool ($1 for children and $2 for adults). The gorge-bottom trail winds past three large waterfalls while climbing up and down stone staircases built

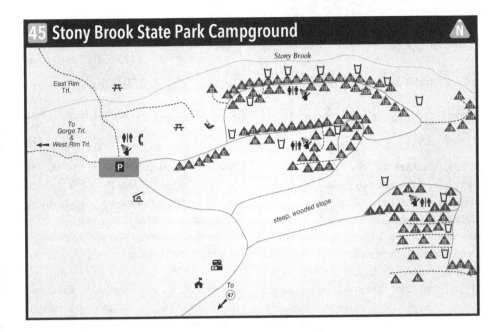

45 Stony Brook State Park Campground

by the Depression-era Civilian Conservation Corps, which also built most of the park's buildings. There are many beautiful gorges in the Finger Lakes region, but few of the region's parks offer as scenic a campground as the one at Stony Brook.

:: Getting There

From I-90 (New York State Thruway), take Exit 46, I-390 South/Corning. Follow I-390 for 43.3 miles to Exit 4, Dansville. Go right on NY 36 South. After 1.2 miles, the main park entrance is on the left. Stay on NY 36 a little more than 1 mile and turn left on CR 47. The campground entrance is on the left.

GPS COORDINATES   N42° 30.683'   W77° 41.817'

46

Taughannock Falls State Park

Taughannock Falls State Park offers all the features that outdoors enthusiasts come to expect of the Finger Lakes.

When visitors to the Finger Lakes think of the region's natural beauty, images of waterfalls, picturesque gorges, and deep glacially cut lakes spring to mind. With a dramatic waterfall, a gorge, and lake access, Taughannock Falls State Park offers all of the features outdoors enthusiasts come to expect of the Finger Lakes. The spectacular waterfall is the centerpiece of the park—at an astounding 215 feet tall, it is the highest free-falling waterfall in the Northeast. You can view it from above at a drive-up overlook as well as from below along a gorge trail that is broad, level, and accessible to most people.

After the last glacial period, glaciers retreated and the waterfall was formed over millennia, as Taughannock Creek flowed over hard Tully limestone and cut away at Sherburne sandstone and Geneseo shale. The erosion process formed a hanging canyon, so the sheer walls at the falls' basin are actually 400 feet high, which makes the basin a very dramatic vantage point. The waters surge in the spring, making the falls truly a wonder, but in summer they die down, so

:: Ratings

BEAUTY: ★ ★ ★
PRIVACY: ★ ★ ★
QUIET: ★ ★ ★
CLEANLINESS: ★ ★ ★
SECURITY: ★ ★
SPACIOUSNESS: ★ ★ ★

visitors may wish to time their trip early in the spring to see the falls in its full majesty. The rocks washed away by Taughannock Creek and over the falls have, over the centuries, formed a delta on Cayuga Lake—today the site of the park's lawn, picnic area, and most of the day-use activities. As in other New York state parks, most of the structures and other park infrastructure are products of work by park staff and the Civilian Conservation Corps during the 1930s.

The campground in Taughannock Falls State Park is located off a public road that leads to the Falls Overlook. The camping area is essentially laid out in a figure eight that runs across a steep hillside. Consequently, a change in elevation as you move around the loop helps to increase privacy throughout the campground. The sites near the entrance are electric, mostly gravel, and obviously favorable for RVs and trailers. At the next part of the figure eight, the sites are designated mostly as tent-only and have larger trees, increased shade, and a denser understory. As you drive through the upper part of the figure eight, the sites are designated as tent and trailer and are consequently very spacious, have ample shade, and some understory.

The road then descends to the lower part of the loop, where you can catch intermittent glimpses of Cayuga Lake through the trees. In summer, the canopy of hardwoods downslope from the campsites obscures the view, but after the leaves drop in fall, there

:: Key Information

ADDRESS: 2221 Taughannock Park Rd., Trumansburg, NY 14886

OPERATED BY: New York State Office of Parks, Recreation and Historic Preservation

CONTACT: 607-387-6739; nysparks.com/parks/62/details.aspx

OPEN: Late April–mid-October

SITES: 74 tent sites, including 16 electric sites

SITE AMENITIES: Picnic table and fire ring

ASSIGNMENT: Choose from available sites or reservations

REGISTRATION: 3 p.m.–9 p.m.

FACILITIES: Picnic areas, pavilions, potable water, flush toilets, snack bar, swimming area, bathhouse, marina, playgrounds, showers

PARKING: At site

FEE: $15/night most tent sites; add $3/night Fridays, Saturdays, and holidays

ELEVATION: 396'

RESTRICTIONS:

■ **Pets:** Dogs on leash with proof of currently valid rabies vaccination

■ **Fires:** In fire rings only

■ **Alcohol:** Allowed

■ **Vehicles:** RVs and trailers limited to specific sites

■ **Other:** Quiet hours 10 p.m.–7 a.m.

■ **Reservations:** 2-night stay required

are open views of the lake. The sites along the exterior here are large, more shaded, and definitely offer the best views in the campground. Quite a few of these sites are tent-only and blend into the large hardwood trees. The interior sites here are smaller, have less shade, are closer together, and have very limited lake views. As the loop approaches the entrance, the sites on both the interior and exterior get smaller and closer together, and their views of the lake become increasingly blocked by the surrounding trees.

Hiking in the park includes the gorge trail, two rim trails, and a multiuse trail. On the park's lawn you'll find multiple picnic areas; fishing is available from the lakeshore and from the fishing pier. Cayuga Lake's fish include lake, brown, and rainbow trout; smallmouth, largemouth, and rock bass; yellow perch; chain pickerel; northern pike; and landlocked salmon. A public boat launch and marina are located south of Taughannock Creek, but note that the park's website indicates that the launch is not suitable for any type of sailboat.

Overnight berths are available by calling the park in advance. Swimming is restricted to a designated area in a protected cove on the south side of the park's lawn area. The park also offers a summer concert series, so campers might want to book their trip to coincide with a favorite performance; call for schedules. A short drive south brings campers to Ithaca and all of its attractions, and to the north and west are some of the popular Finger Lakes wine trails.

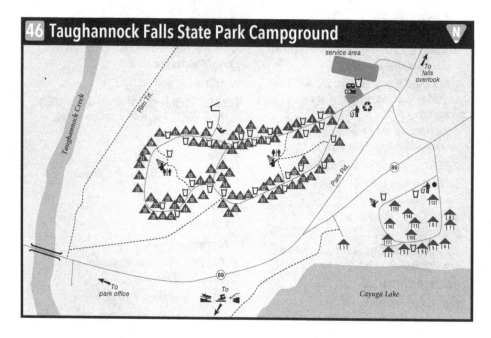

:: Getting There

From I-81 South, take Exit 12, NY 281/Cortland. Stay left on the exit ramp until you reach the stop sign. Turn left on NY 281 and follow it 3.8 miles. NY 281 becomes NY 13; continue on NY 13 for 21 miles through Dryden into Ithaca. Turn right on West Buffalo Street/NY 89/NY 96, then right again on NY 89. Follow NY 89 for 9.3 miles to the park entrance, on the right.

GPS COORDINATES   N42° 32.733'   W76° 35.900'

47

Watkins Glen State Park

With its plunging waterfalls and water-sculpted rock, the gorge of Watkins Glen is a wondrous combination of artificial and natural beauty.

On the southern shores of Seneca Lake lies one of the most spectacular gorges in the Finger Lakes region. With its hand-cut tunnels, arched bridges, winding stone staircases, water-drilled pools, 19 plunging waterfalls, and water-sculpted rock, the 400-foot gorge of Watkins Glen is a wondrous combination of artificial and naturally carved beauty.

During the 19th century, the glen was operated as a tourist resort until New York State purchased this marvel in 1906. The Gorge Trail explores the interior of the gorge, and you can visit the rim via the Indian and South Rim Trails. In fact, the South Rim Trail forms a part of both the Finger Lakes Trail and the North Country National Scenic Trail. The Finger Lakes Trail traverses part of southern and western New York, connecting the Catskill Mountains with Allegany State Park; the North Country NST, when completed, will connect Lake Champlain in New York with Lake Sakakawea in North Dakota.

:: Ratings

BEAUTY: ★ ★
PRIVACY: ★ ★ ★
QUIET: ★ ★ ★
CLEANLINESS: ★ ★ ★
SECURITY: ★ ★ ★ ★
SPACIOUSNESS: ★ ★ ★

Less-ambitious hikers or those with time constraints should hike the Gorge Trail as a round-trip, or take advantage of a park shuttle bus to return to the main parking area.

The campground's six "villages," or loops, are named after various American Indian tribes that have inhabited New York State: Cayuga, Mohawk, Oneida, Onondaga, Seneca, and Tuscarora. Almost all the sites are densely forested; each loop has a comfort station and multiple Dumpsters.

Although Cayuga Village (sites 1–49) has a similar number of sites as the other loops, it is slightly smaller, and consequently the sites are less spacious and closer together. Large red pines thoroughly shade the area, but there is very little understory, leaving the sites visible to each other. Even less private are the sites (odd numbers 27–37, and 38) that back up to Mohawk Village and the 10 sites (39–49) situated directly on a road that serves two of the loops.

The neighboring loop, Mohawk Village (sites 50–105), contains the only electric sites in the campground, which cost more than those in other loops. The initial sites are closest to Cayuga Village, are quite large, and lie a little higher than the rest of the loop. These sites are best suited to larger RVs and contain all of the higher-amp electric sites. Near the loop's eastern edge, the

:: Key Information

ADDRESS: Route 14, Watkins Glen, NY 14891

OPERATED BY: New York State Office of Parks, Recreation and Historic Preservation

CONTACT: 607-535-4511; nysparks .com/parks/142/details.aspx

OPEN: Mid-May–early October

SITES: 305 sites, including 54 electric sites

SITE AMENITIES: Picnic table and fire ring

ASSIGNMENT: Choose from available sites or reservations

REGISTRATION: 3 p.m.–9 p.m.

FACILITIES: Picnic areas, pavilion, potable water, flush toilets, park store, swimming pool, showers

PARKING: At site

FEE: $15 (Oneida Village) $19/night most other tent sites (plus $4/night on Fridays, Saturdays, and holidays)

ELEVATION: 726'

RESTRICTIONS:

▪ **Pets:** Dogs on leash with proof of currently valid rabies vaccination

▪ **Fires:** In fire rings only

▪ **Alcohol:** Allowed

▪ **Vehicles:** RVs and trailers limited to specific sites

▪ **Other:** Quiet hours 10 p.m.–7 a.m.

▪ **Reservations:** 2-night stay required; 1-night reservations available if reserved within 7 days of visit

road descends, providing wooded views of Seneca Lake. The change in elevation makes this area far more removed from the rest of the village—but the understory remains sparse, and the sites here are still visible to each other. Given the increased cost, tent campers might want to look elsewhere—but since these are the only views of the lake, take a peek to see what is available.

Nestled in the center of the entire campground is Oneida Village (sites 106–153), which, incidentally, offers the most affordable sites. A canopy of pines and hardwoods shades the area, and a dense understory and multiple changes in terrain lead to a wide variety of site sizes. Not surprisingly, most of the sites here are designated as tent-only—since the sites are considerably more private than in the previous villages, campers seeking seclusion and who don't require much space should give this area a good look.

The next two villages, Onondaga and Seneca, are off a short access road but are separate enough not to neighbor each other. Sites within Onondaga Village (154–203) are generally large and shady—the notable exceptions being sites 185–188, which lie on a lawn and are very public. The initial sites along this loop have dense saplings between them and are tent-only. The sites get larger and more spread out near the loop's midpoint, with sites along the periphery extending farthest into the surrounding forest. Seneca Village (sites 204–251) is similar to Onondaga, but because its loop is larger, the sites are more spread out and feel more remote. Tall hardwoods shade all of the sites here, and some understory is present throughout. A deep woodland setting generally characterizes these two loops, with plenty of good options for tent campers.

The last village, Tuscarora (sites 252–305), encircles a large lawn that contains a

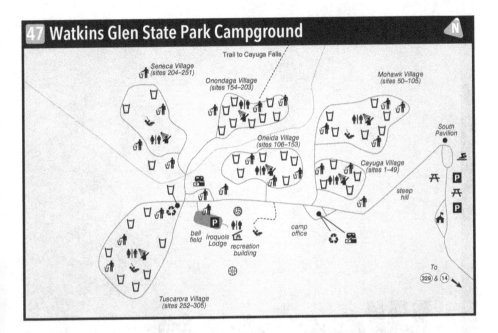

47 Watkins Glen State Park Campground

playground—but since this loop is much larger than previous ones, the sites are more spread out. Although many sites along the interior either back up to or lie upon the lawn area, some of the park's best sites are found here. The first dozen are similar to those in Oneida Village, since they have dense undergrowth and are fairly shallow. Near site 265, interior sites sprawl into the encircled lawn and peripheral sites extend back into the forest. Sites on the perimeter are tent-only, their dense vegetation and depth providing some seclusion. Interior sites revert to a woodland setting at site 276, but beyond site 283, sites on both sides of the road open up to the lawn. The sites again revert to a woodland setting at sites 291 and 294, but these are far more closely spaced than other wooded sites in the loop. The last few lie next to the loop's entrance and consequently are not very private or desirable.

Visitors to the park should be aware that the annual Watkins Glen International NASCAR races, held each summer, result in solid bookings for a week or more at this and every other nearby campground.

:: Getting There

From I-90 (New York State Thruway), take Exit 42, NY 14/Geneva/Lyons. Follow NY 14 South 42.4 miles through most of the village of Watkins Glen. The main park entrance is on the right.

GPS COORDINATES   N42° 22.550'   W76° 52.267'

Western
New York

48

Allegany State Park:

Cain Hollow (Quaker Area)

Untouched by Ice Age glaciers, the landscape, topography, and geology of Allegany State Park are quite different from what most New Yorkers are used to.

At 65,000 acres, Allegany State Park is the largest state park in New York. Considering that the park borders Pennsylvania's Allegheny National Forest, which covers more than 500,000 acres, this area is truly a vast wilderness. This wilderness park is unique for two reasons: first, unlike the Adirondacks and Catskills, it is a state park, not a state forest; and second, the area was unglaciated. Glacial influences on the landscape are evident across all of New York except, for all practical purposes, within the boundaries of this park. Untouched by Ice Age glaciers, the landscape, topography, and geology of Allegany State Park are quite different from what most New Yorkers are used to. This unglaciated area, called the Salamanca Reentrant, consists of terrain that is more angular and rugged than the deeply gouged troughs and subdued terrain found in the rest of the state. Established in 1921 to provide the western half of New York with its own "wilderness playground," the park is a great destination for campers wishing to vary their wilderness experiences in New York.

The park consists of two main sections, the Red House Area to the north and the Quaker Area to the south. Within these two sections are 375 cabins (the actual number available varies from year to year and season to season) and three camping areas: the Cain Hollow Camping Area, the Red House Tent and Trailer Area, and the Diehl Tent and Trailer Trail. Located in the Quaker Area, the Diehl campsites are intermixed with cabins and are not particularly desirable, unless part of your camping party wishes to stay in cabins. The Red House Area, with a total of 139 tent and RV sites, has a densely wooded section (Loops B–E) with sites that vary widely in size, spacing, and privacy, as well as an open field area (Loop A) containing more-public (and less-desirable) sites. Although there are many good sites in the Red House Area, the nonelectric sites at Cain Hollow, described following, are prime choices for the tent camper.

Also located in the Quaker Area (and sometimes referred to by that name outside the park), Cain Hollow is divided into two main groups: sites 1–42 and sites 43–164. The first group lies on an open field without any trees or privacy—but since these all have 50-amp electric hookups, they are more suitable for trailers and RVs. The second group

:: Ratings

BEAUTY: ★ ★
PRIVACY: ★ ★ ★ ★
QUIET: ★ ★ ★
CLEANLINESS: ★ ★ ★
SECURITY: ★ ★ ★ ★
SPACIOUSNESS: ★ ★ ★

:: Key Information

ADDRESS: Cain Hollow Rd., Salamanca, NY 14779

OPERATED BY: New York State Office of Parks, Recreation and Historic Preservation

CONTACT: 716-354-2182; nysparks .com/parks/1/details.aspx

OPEN: Memorial Day–Columbus Day (Cain Hollow Camping Area)

SITES: 164 tent sites, including 133 electric sites

SITE AMENITIES: Picnic table and fire ring

ASSIGNMENT: Choose from available sites or reservations

REGISTRATION: 3 p.m.–9 p.m.

FACILITIES: Picnic areas, pavilion, potable water, flush toilets, park store, boat launch, museums, showers

PARKING: At site

FEE: $15/night most tent sites; $6–$8/ night additional for sites with electric hookups (extra $4/night on Fridays, Saturdays, and holidays)

ELEVATION: 1,453'

RESTRICTIONS:

■ **Pets:** Dogs on leash with proof of currently valid rabies vaccination

■ **Fires:** In fire rings only

■ **Alcohol:** Allowed

■ **Vehicles:** RVs and trailers allowed

■ **Other:** Quiet hours 10 p.m.–8 a.m.

■ **Reservations:** 2-night stay required; 1-night reservations available if reserved within 3 days of visit

has a central road that serves several spur roads and loops, which interweave into one another but eventually rejoin the central road.

The numbering system is a bit confusing, as roads and loops seem to bisect each other and numbers run counterclockwise and clockwise in different sections. The only real way to figure out why you are now at site 121 after having driven past, say, site 79 is to look at a map. The entire group is on a hill, and the changes in elevation help increase the privacy throughout. Although the sites higher up yield partially obscured views into the sites below, the lower sites can't see into the sites above them at all. Consequently, the most private sites lie on the upper part of the hill. Coincidentally, these sites (140–164) are also among the most spacious in the group, making them the best choice for campers who wish for a little more solitude. Sites 96–109 and 131–139, on

the hill's northeastern edge, are grassy and quite open, with little shade. The interior sites (74–95 and 120–130) are shady, well sized, and surrounded with brush, making them private and a good choice for most tent campers. The exceptions are sites 110–119, which are fairly open.

Bordering the main access road are two groups of very shady sites. Sites 43–55 are close together and fairly public. Sites 56–73 are more spread out and have a denser understory; many are by a creek. These sites are a good choice, but their electric hookups and designation as prime sites make them more expensive. During the winter of 2013, the electric service for the campground was upgraded. Sites 1–80 and 120–123 will have 50-amp services ($8 additional per night). Sites 81–102, 104–119, and 124–134 have 30-amp services ($6 additional per night). The remaining sites are nonelectric and best suited for tent campers.

48 Allegany State Park Campground: Cain Hollow (Quaker Area)

Fortunately these were and are the most desirable sites for tent campers.

Though most of this park can be considered wilderness, it also contains pockets of development more akin to small villages than typical park facilities. Indeed, this seems to have been the logic behind dividing the park into two sections, as the Red House and Quaker areas are the two hubs of development. The colonies of cabins often resemble neighborhoods on the fringes of each village's cluster of stores, museums, and dining and recreational venues.

Because the park is so large, bringing a bike (rentals are available) is a good idea. Miles of hiking trails allow campers to explore the mixed-hardwood forests, mountains, streams, and ponds. Two artificial lakes offer swimming at sandy beaches and boating activities. To ensure quiet, calm waters, boating is limited to nonmotorized craft or boats with only small motors. Visitors who wish to gain a deeper understanding of the park's history and natural features can join the park staff and naturalists on structured tours, walks, or similar activities. The park is open year-round—numerous winterized cabins allow visitors to explore this wilderness by ski, snowshoe, or snowmobile.

:: Getting There

From I-86, take Exit 18, NY 280. Head south on NY 280 for 4.4 miles. The park entrance is straight ahead.

GPS COORDINATES   N42° 02.733'   W78°52.267'

49

Lakeside Beach State Park

Sites along the middle of Loops A, B, C, and D lie very close to the lake, and the sounds of water lapping on its rocky shore are particularly pleasant here.

The Great Lakes contain 20% of the world's surface fresh water—a staggering fact in and of itself—but more pertinent is the lakes' continual influence on the region's environment, most notably through lake-effect rain and snow, a constant source of grumbling in central New York. Within the immediate vicinity of the Great Lakes, winds blowing off the lakes create a more favorable environment for agriculture—which explains why the southern shores of Lake Ontario contain some of New York's most productive fruit orchards. Nestled among these orchards is Lakeside Beach State Park. In fact, up until 1962, when the state established the 743-acre park, it was farmland and fruit orchards.

The campground is laid out in seven one-way loops, with the first four bordering Lake Ontario. The loops in this pet-free area (A, B, C, and D) are laid out roughly the same and share similar characteristics. The first and last couple of sites along each

of these loops lie on an open lawn, which leaves campers plenty of room to spread out but not much privacy. The forested areas have a dense tree canopy as well as shrubs, saplings, and other vegetation, all of which enhance the woodland feel and increase privacy as well. The amply sized sites are a little closely spaced, but the understory prevents the area from feeling crowded. Sites along the middle of the loops lie very close to the lake, and the sounds of water lapping on its rocky shore are particularly pleasant here. Although many of the park's sites are similar, campers will want to take note of some differences. For example, Loop A is wooded only along its initial third (sites 4–13). The rest of the sites lie on an open lawn with only a few shade trees interspersed. Though these sites lack the seclusion characteristic of those in the forest, they do have the benefit of fine views of the lake. Although sites in the loop's center and closer to its end have poor views, those at the lake's edge (14–23) have truly expansive views of Lake Ontario. Clearly, the peripheral sites are the primary choice along this loop.

Along the other loops, the views of the lake, where available, are generally thinly veiled by the surrounding forest—though this is really an enhancement rather than a detraction. On Loop B, lake views begin around site 19 and conclude around site

:: Ratings

BEAUTY: ★ ★ ★
PRIVACY: ★ ★ ★
QUIET: ★ ★ ★
CLEANLINESS: ★ ★ ★
SECURITY: ★ ★ ★
SPACIOUSNESS: ★ ★ ★

:: Key Information

ADDRESS: NY 18, Waterport, NY 14571

OPERATED BY: New York State Office of Parks, Recreation and Historic Preservation

CONTACT: 585-682-4888; nysparks .com/parks/161/details.aspx

OPEN: Early May–Mid October

SITES: 274 tent sites, all electric

SITE AMENITIES: Picnic table and fire ring

ASSIGNMENT: Choose from available sites or reservations

REGISTRATION: 3 p.m.–9 p.m.

FACILITIES: Picnic areas, potable water, flush toilets, park store, laundry, showers

PARKING: At site

FEE: $21 or $27/night (plus $4/night on Fridays, Saturdays, and holidays)

ELEVATION: 289'

RESTRICTIONS:

■ **Pets:** Limited to Loops E, F, and G; dogs on leash with proof of currently valid rabies vaccination

■ **Fires:** In fire rings only

■ **Alcohol:** Allowed

■ **Vehicles:** RVs and trailers allowed

■ **Other:** Quiet hours 10 p.m.–7 a.m.

■ **Reservations:** 2-night stay required; 1-night reservations available if reserved within 3 days of visit

28—these are also some of the best sites in the whole campground. On Loop C, Lake Ontario reveals itself around site 17 and disappears around site 28. On Loop D, the lake becomes visible around site 7 because of a neighboring lawn and playing field; the views become really magnificent around site 12 but then decline at site 20, where the thick woodlands come to dominate the landscape. Sites beside the lawn are a little less private, since the forest is fairly thin—but the added views are fair compensation. Whether forested or open, sites in this part of the campground provide sounds and smells of the lake that are particularly appealing.

The next area, which includes all of the loops that allow pets (E–G), lies across the road from the park store, laundry, recreation hall, and playfield. Loop E begins and ends with seven sites (1–4 and 39–41) that have views of Lake Ontario down and across the playfield. These spacious lawn sites are wide open, with no shade. Dense conifers and shrubs to the south and east enclose this section, which ends after site 22, where the loop enters the forest. Within the forest, the sites have less understory, so there is more room to spread out than in the previous forested sites bordering the lake. Also, the woodland sites have a more open-woodland feel, as beech and its telltale thickets become the dominant species. Loop E reverts to a lawn setting at site 38, but more woodland sites are available along Loop F.

All of the sites on Loop F are within forest, with the exception of 23–31, which are on a lawn. Glimpses of Lake Ontario are available from sites 1, 3, 5, and 6, making these scenic choices for pet owners whose choices are limited to these loops. Loop G is composed entirely of wide-open lawn sites exactly like those along Loop E, only without lake views.

Although there is no swimming beach or boat launch within the park, the lakeside setting nevertheless provides an excellent camping choice. Visitors who wish to boat on Lake Ontario can launch at Oak Orchard

State Park, a short drive east along Orchard Creek. Camping registration gives you access to this boat launch. Excellent fishing is available along the creek and in Lake Ontario.

:: Getting There

From I-90 (New York State Thruway), take Exit 48, NY 98/Batavia. Head north along NY 98 toward Albion and continue 24 miles. Merge straight ahead onto NY 18, follow it 2.5 miles, and then turn right onto Lakeside Beach Road. The park entrance is straight ahead.

GPS COORDINATES   N43° 22.000'   W78° 14.150'

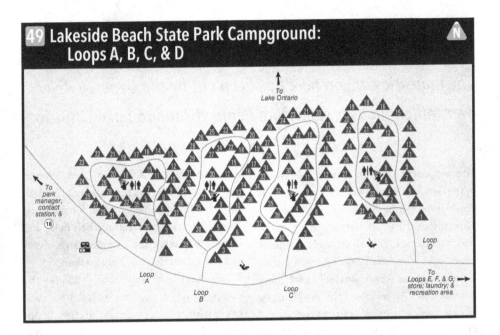

49 Lakeside Beach State Park Campground: Loops A, B, C, & D

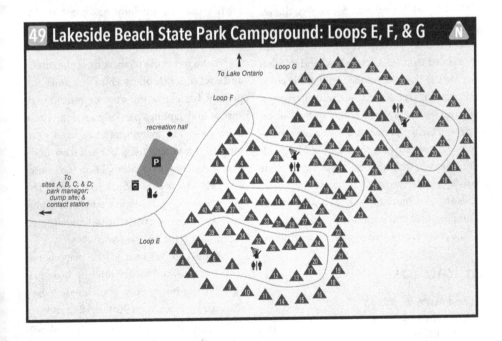

49 Lakeside Beach State Park Campground: Loops E, F, & G

50

Letchworth State Park

The majestic canyon here has been cut by the Genesee River over millennia as it runs from Pennsylvania to Lake Ontario.

The majestic canyon here has been cut by the Genesee River over millennia as it runs north from Pennsylvania to Lake Ontario. Throughout the park, dramatic views of the sheer sandstone and shale walls, some of which rise more than 600 feet, are visible from numerous scenic overlooks and along the popular Gorge Trail. The park's three large waterfalls are visible from the trail, the tallest of which, Middle Falls, drops 107 feet and is illuminated each night May–October.

The park is very well developed, thanks to its namesake, William Pryor Letchworth, who originally purchased 190 acres and then proceeded to acquire more land and develop the area so that the public could easily enjoy this natural wonder. Extensive construction was carried out by the Civilian Conservation Corps, which expanded upon the infrastructure. A truly striking example of the work done here is the arched stone bridge that crosses the Genesee River below the Lower Falls at a very dramatic flume. The Highbanks Camping Area and swimming pools are some of the more recent and significant additions.

:: Ratings

BEAUTY: ★ ★
PRIVACY: ★ ★ ★
QUIET: ★ ★
CLEANLINESS: ★ ★ ★
SECURITY: ★ ★ ★ ★ ★
SPACIOUSNESS: ★ ★ ★

The Highbanks Camping Area is separated from the rest of the park by a check-in area that limits vehicle access. A park store, laundry, recreation building, ball field, and playground serve the camping area. Every site has a minimum 20-amp hookup.

Several one-way loops divide the campground; these run parallel to each other within their respective groups. Loops 100 and 200 form one group; Loops 300–600 form a second, and Loops 700 and 800 form a third. Each loop has comfort stations with showers, a recycling station, and a Dumpster.

Loop 100 is the farthest from the others and consequently offers a bit more quiet and privacy. Generally, the sites are roomy, with shrubs and saplings partially masking them from view. The exterior sites at the beginning of Loop 100 neighbor sites on Loop 200, but sites farther along Loop 100's outer edge blend into the hardwood forest. The inner sites along this loop are more spacious but have less cover, with the last few situated essentially upon an open lawn.

Loop 200 lies next to the playground, with a sparse understory offering little privacy for the initial edge sites. These grassy sites are denser, have less shade, and are openly visible to each other. The southern edge of this loop offers the most privacy, with ample shade from the forest canopy. The last few sites along the edge of Loop 200 abut the road, and openings in the understory reveal

:: Key Information

ADDRESS: 1 Letchworth State Park, Castile, NY 14427

OPERATED BY: New York State Office of Parks, Recreation and Historic Preservation

CONTACT: 585-237-3303; nysparks .com/parks/79/details.aspx

OPEN: Mid-May–mid-October

SITES: 270 tent sites, all electric

SITE AMENITIES: Picnic table and fire ring

ASSIGNMENT: Choose from available sites or reservations

REGISTRATION: 3 p.m.–9 p.m.

FACILITIES: Picnic areas, pavilion, potable water, flush toilets, showers, laundry, ball field, playgrounds, pool, museum, inn and restaurant

PARKING: At site

FEE: $21/night most tent sites (plus $4/night on Fridays, Saturdays, and holidays)

ELEVATION: 919'

RESTRICTIONS:

■ **Pets:** Limited to Loops 100, 200, and 700 only; dogs on leash with proof of currently valid rabies vaccination

■ **Fires:** In fire rings only

■ **Alcohol:** Allowed

■ **Vehicles:** 1 RV or trailer per site

■ **Other:** Quiet hours 10 p.m.–7 a.m.

■ **Reservations:** 2-night stay required; 1-night reservations available if reserved within 3 days of visit

vehicle traffic as well as bike and foot traffic heading to the trailheads near the beginning of Loop 100.

Loops 300, 400, 500, and 600 are all very similar to each other: they are all roughly elongated ovals running from their entrances on the western end toward undisturbed forests to the east. The ellipses are essentially parallel, so that sites along the longer sides back up to one another. Consequently, sites at the eastern end are the most spacious and private, and therefore the most desirable. Generally speaking, the interior sites are smaller, less shaded, and more public, as they are usually closest to the central comfort station. All of the sites would be considered in the forest and have increasing amounts of shade the farther you get from the interior of these loops.

Loop 300 borders the ball field; sites on the loop's northern edge are on an open lawn beside the field, and so are highly visible to the public. On Loop 400, sites are generally more spacious and shady and have some understory between them, which makes them a little more private than others within this group. On Loop 500, sites have fewer shrubs than on previous loops, but many are also shadier and have grassy areas. The last loop, 600, is separated from the steep banks along its southern edge by a chain-link fence. Its sites are more removed from the public areas of the campground and have only one neighboring loop, but a lack of shrubs makes them more visible to each other than on other loops.

Loops 700 and 800 are closest to the campground entrance and have some of the largest sites. These loops are also composed of elongated ovals running parallel to each other, though in this case their orientation is north–south, with entrances to the north and woods to the south. Not surprisingly, the south end is the shadiest and most spacious.

The long sides of Loop 700 are visible either to Loop 800 or to the road that provides access to the previous group. Multiple sites on Loop 700 are lawn sites and have 50-amp hookups, so the area is best suited to large RVs. Sites on Loop 800 are similar to those on Loop 700 in that they are deep and seem suited to RVs. However, sites along the southern edge of Loop 800 border the woods, enjoy plenty of shade, and have a lush understory.

The park's developed areas include numerous picnic grounds as well as two swimming pools, cabins, a lodge, an inn, a restaurant, concession stands, a museum, and several historic sites. Winding roads lead you through beautiful hardwood forests crisscrossed by hiking trails. Private outfitters within the park's boundaries offer daily hot-air-balloon rides along the river, horseback riding, and canoeing and rafting trips.

:: Getting There

From I-90 (New York State Thruway), take Exit 46, I-390 South/Corning. Follow I-390 for 27.2 miles to Exit 7, NY 408/Mount Morris/Letchworth State Park. Turn left onto NY 408/Mount Morris Geneseo Road and follow it 1.8 miles. Turn right on NY 36/Main Street; go north for 1.1 miles. The park entrance is on the left.

GPS COORDINATES N42° 44.417' W77° 53.433'

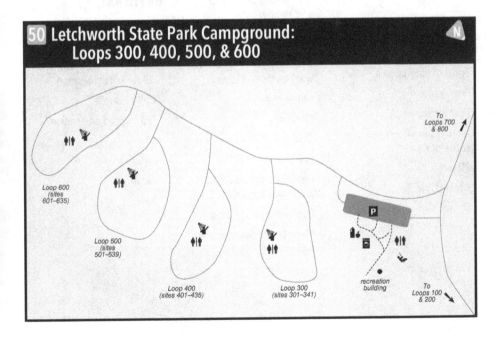

APPENDIX A

• •

Camping-Equipment Checklist

You may want to keep a plastic storage container full of the essentials for car camping, so they're ready to go when you are. Then you can make a last-minute check of the inventory, resupply anything that's low or missing, and away you go. Here's a reminder list:

COOKING UTENSILS

Aluminum foil

Bottle opener

Bottles of salt, pepper, spices, sugar, cooking oil, and maple syrup in water-proof, spill-proof containers

Can opener

Cups, plastic or metal

Dish-washing soap (*biodegradable*), sponge, and towel

Flatware

Food of your choice

Frying pan

Fuel for stove

Matches in waterproof container

Plates

Pocketknife

Pot with lid

Spatula

Stove

Wooden spoon

FIRST-AID KIT

(See Introduction, page 5, for a complete list.)

SLEEPING GEAR

Pillow

Sleeping bag

Sleeping pad, inflatable or insulated

Tent with ground tarp and rainfly

MISCELLANEOUS

Bath soap (*biodegradable*), washcloth, and towel

Camp chair

Candles

Cooler

Fire starter

Flashlight or headlamp with fresh batteries

Foul-weather clothing

Maps (road, topographic, trail, etc.)

Paper towels

Plastic zip-top bags

Playing cards

Sunglasses

Toilet paper

Trowel (for burying solid waste)

Water bottle

Wool blanket

OPTIONAL

Barbecue grill

Binoculars

Books on bird, plant, and wildlife identification

Cell phone

Fishing rod and tackle

GPS

Hatchet

Lantern

Saw

APPENDIX B

Sources of Information

ADIRONDACK MOUNTAIN CLUB
814 Goggins Rd.
Lake George, NY 12845
518-668-4447
adk.org

**ADIRONDACK
REGIONAL TOURISM COUNCIL**
P.O. Box 911
Lake Placid, NY 12946
518-846-8016
visitadirondacks.com

APPALACHIAN MOUNTAIN CLUB
5 Joy St.
Boston, MA 02108
617-523-0655
outdoors.org

**APPALACHIAN TRAIL CONSERVANCY,
MID-ATLANTIC REGIONAL OFFICE**
4 E. 1st St.
Boiling Springs, PA 17007
717-258-5771
appalachiantrail.org

CATSKILL MOUNTAIN CLUB
P.O. Box 558
Pine Hill, NY 12465
catskillmountainclub.org

FINGER LAKES TRAIL CONFERENCE
6111 Visitor Center Rd.
Mt. Morris, NY 14510
585-658-9320
fingerlakestrail.org

**NATIONAL PARK SERVICE,
FIRE ISLAND NATIONAL SEASHORE**
120 Laurel St.
Patchogue, NY 11772
631-697-4750
nps.gov/fiis

**NEW YORK STATE DEPARTMENT
OF ECONOMIC DEVELOPMENT-
NEW YORK STATE TOURISM**
800-225-5697
iloveny.com

**NEW YORK STATE DEPARTMENT OF
ENVIRONMENTAL CONSERVATION**
625 Broadway
Albany, NY 12233
518-402-8013
www.dec.ny.gov

**NEW YORK STATE OFFICE OF
PARKS, RECREATION &
HISTORIC PRESERVATION**
625 Broadway
Albany NY, 12207
518-237-8643
nysparks.com

**NEW YORK WINE &
GRAPE FOUNDATION**
800 S. Main St., Ste. 200
Canandaigua, NY 14424
585-394-3620
newyorkwines.org

**NORTH COUNTRY TRAIL
ASSOCIATION**
229 E. Main St.
Lowell, MI 49331
866-445-3628
northcountrytrail.org

NORTHERN FOREST CANOE TRAIL
P.O. Box 565
Waitsfield, VT 05673
802-496-2285
northernforestcanoetrail.org

RESERVEAMERICA
800-456-2267, **reserveamerica.com**

APPENDIX B

● ●

Sources of Information *(continued)*

SEAWAY TRAIL
P.O. Box 660
401 W. Main St.
Sackets Harbor, NY 13685
315-646-1000
seawaytrail.com

SUFFOLK COUNTY DEPARTMENT OF PARKS, RECREATION AND CONSERVATION
P.O. Box 6100
100 Veterans Memorial Hwy.
Hauppauge, NY 11788
631-853-5593
suffolkcountyny.gov

APPENDIX C

Suggested Reading and Reference

Bailey, Bill. *New York State Parks: A Complete Outdoor Recreation Guide.* Glovebox Books of America, 1997.

Burdick, Neal S. (Series Ed.). *Guide to Adirondack Trails* (Volumes 1–7). Adirondack Mountain Club, 1993–2004.

Cooper, James Fenimore. *The Leatherstocking Tales* (Volumes 1–2). Library of America, 1995.

Ehling, William. *50 Hikes in Central New York.* Countryman Press, 1995.

Ehling, William. *50 Hikes in Western New York.* Countryman Press, 1990.

Folwell, Elizabeth. *The Adirondack Book.* Berkshire House Publishers, 2003.

Hartman, Gary. *The Campgrounds of New York.* New Country Books, 2007.

Irving, Washington. *History, Tales, and Sketches.* Library of America, 1983.

Kick, Peter. *Catskill Mountain Guide.* Appalachian Mountain Club, 2009.

Lewis, Tom. *The Hudson: A History.* Yale University Press, 2007.

McKibben, Bill. *Wandering Home: A Long Walk Across America's Most Hopeful Landscape—Vermont's Champlain Valley and New York's Adirondacks.* Crown, 2005.

McMartin, Barbara. *50 Hikes in the Adirondacks.* Countryman Press, 2003.

Ostertag, Rhonda and George. *Hiking New York.* FalconGuides, 2009.

Schneider, Paul. *The Adirondacks: A History of America's First Wilderness.* Holt Paperbacks, 1998.

Starmer, Timothy. *Five-Star Trails in the Adirondacks.* Menasha Ridge Press, 2010.

Starmer, Timothy. *Five-Star Trails in the Finger Lakes and Central New York.* Menasha Ridge Press, 2013.

Trails Illustrated Maps. *Adirondack Park* series (Maps 742–746) and *Catskill Park* (Map 755). National Geographic, 2011–2013.

Van Diver, Bradford B. *Roadside Geology of New York.* Mountain Press Publishing Company, 1985.

INDEX

ABOUT THE AUTHORS

Growing up outside of Syracuse, **Aaron Starmer** spent his childhood exploring the wilds of central New York. As a present for graduating from Drew University, he received a tent, which has become his favorite accommodation on trips around the country. He has pitched it on the rim of the Grand Canyon, in the shadow of the Watchman at Zion National Park, deep in the woods of the Great Smoky Mountains, and on Flamenco Beach in Culebra, Puerto Rico. He is a contributor to numerous guidebooks on New York and the author of novels for children, including *DWEEB, The Only Ones,* and the upcoming *The Riverman.* He lives in Hoboken, New Jersey, with his wife (and coauthor), Cate, and daughter, Hannah.

Cate Starmer was born on Cape Cod, and her parents' many moves throughout the Northeast inspired her lifelong wanderlust. She pitched her first tent as a Girl Scout in Penn's Woods. Backpacking trips during college took her as far as Australia, Thailand, and Costa Rica. Her favorite camping spots are usually near the water, such as in New Zealand's Abel Tasman Park, along the Colorado River in the Grand Canyon, and Watch Hill on Fire Island. Currently working for Fodor's Travel in New York City, Cate often loads up her pack and escapes into the wilderness on weekends with coauthor (and husband) Aaron—though admittedly she likes hiking in to backcountry huts as much as she likes car camping. She always makes sure her first-aid kit contains heaps of bandages, plenty of sunscreen, plus a corkscrew for emergencies.

Timothy Starmer has always been an outdoors enthusiast and spent most of his childhood seeking out remote and wild areas whenever possible. During a brief hiatus from Brown University during 1997, he drove across the United States for six weeks, camping the entire way. Along the route, he explored many of the West's national and state parks, including Canyonlands, Yellowstone, Arches, and Bryce Canyon. He even braved pitching a tent among the mosquito swarms in Badlands National Park. At the trip's conclusion, he headed down to Australia, where he backpacked for a few months exploring

the eastern Outback, the Great Barrier Reef, and the caves of Tasmania, as well as traversing the Tasmanian World Heritage Area along the Overland Track. Tim owns and operates New Heritage Woodworking, a construction company that specializes in designing and building timber frames. But he can still be found exploring the wilds whenever possible.

Printed in the USA
CPSIA information can be obtained
at www.ICGtesting.com
JSHW060928260124
55822JS00007B/19